YOU WERE CREATED FOR GREATNESS

A Philosophy on Wholeness

Jackson Hale

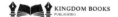 KINGDOM BOOKS
PUBLISHING

Kingdom Books LLC
www.kingdombookspublishing.com

Gratitude

To all who helped, encouraged, and enlightened me along the way, I could not have written this without you. Thank you to my mother and father, my sister, and my brothers and sisters in Christ: Clarence, Tyler, Jamal, Natalie, Tom, Max, Dillon, Carlos, Nick, Becca, Paul, Bryan, Dave, Chad, Julie, Joe, Cassidy, Jeff, Hal, Dan, Shawn, Craig, Mike, Cynthia, Pastor Joel, Brianna, Alyssa, Amanda, Andrea, Dominick, and Professor Crowell. I thank God for the opportunity to present you these next pages, and I give Him all the glory.

I have poured all I know and believe into this book. I pray it produces the good fruit I intend to plant in doing so. Throughout the total 7 chapters, there will be practical questions with the opportunity to explore your current health and wellness. I encourage you to bring a notebook along for the journey and journal what you feel led to. Thank you for reading; it is truly a blessing, and I am honored.

Table of Contents

Preface

Mark 10:43-45 AMP, *"But this is not how it is among you; instead, whoever wishes to become great among you must be your servant, and whoever wishes to be first and most important among you must be slave of all. For even the Son of Man did not come to be served, but to serve, and to give His life as a ransom for many."*

Greatness isn't about money. It isn't about skill. It isn't about the number of people you reach. *It's about the depth of impact one makes in the lives of others.* Through Christ-centered wellness, you can consistently maximize your impact in this world. It will take time, effort, persistence, and focus, but everyone has what it takes. I believe it. After all, we were made in His image.

Now that you host the Holy Spirit as a Believer, you have everything you need. God can use you for His glory. Yet, you have free choice to either cultivate a healthy environment in your life where you can be used to your full potential or squander the opportunity by giving into the temptations and distractions of this world.

You must ask yourself. Which will it be?

Through greatness you will achieve much. Your actions, however, must be tactical and intentional in this world as a Believer. It's needed even more now than ever to be sober minded and full of love in the freedom Christ has given us. God's hope and intention is for you to live your best life for His glory, impacting those in your sphere of influence through His love and power. *Our potential is in Him.*

1

So, you have a path. You have a destiny. Will you say, *"yes"* to a life of wholeness and run your best?

My goal with this book is to pour out everything I have learned, my heart, and what I believe in as a faith-based wellness professional. This is something I now know I need for my own life. God has put it on my heart to write out my belief on personal wholeness, and I have written these pages to piece together what I have found to be essential for consistent health in my life. Please know I am walking this out daily, and I am with you.

I am no expert, doctor, or pastor, but what I do carry is a burning passion to see the body of Christ consistently walk with confidence, power, and love in the Spirit. I am talking about working toward consistent transformation into who He has created you to be!

I don't see physical health as an end-all-be-all. Through personal experience, and helping clients along their own journey, I strongly believe this to be true: there is a deeper health a person needs, and as a Christian myself, I've noticed the Church— His body— needs as well. I have learned in my own life that, as a Believer, you must be diligent and intentional in how you take care of your body, mind, and spirit as you seek to improve, grow, and remain consistent in your walk with God.

You are a complex human being with a great destiny through Christ. However, you have free will. There is opposition, along with many distractions and false truths, in this world constantly pulling you away from your potential. This book will teach you how to build stability in your life, cut through the distractions this world so tangibly holds, and empower your best self to unlock your God-given potential within.

Again, through greatness you will achieve much. Each of your dreams may look different, but no matter where you are in your life, you have value, and you can have a positive impact in the lives of others. It's not what you do but how you do it that makes a difference. *God can use you wherever He plants you, but in order to consistently do your best, you must cultivate and set the foundation for greatness with what I call true wellness, or holistic wholeness in your life.* Amen.

You must realize the Gospel is a holistic message. It brings everlasting life for all who will drink the water of Christ (John 4:12). By letting it seep into every part of your life, you can transform into a new creation. The old is gone. The new is living, and all that held you back in the past is now nothing but a memory (Hebrews 8:11-12). When you step into this truth and trust the scriptures, your identity will begin to come into view. Your true identity. That you are a child of God.

Through this truth, you can begin to love in opposition of the world's selfish and destructive culture, from the way you engage others, to the way you eat, to the way you approach health, and even fitness. *My mission is to bring you into a place of realization of who you are, what you are worth, and the potential of impact you carry for God's kingdom!*

This deep, Christ-centered, holistic take on wellness is my passion for all whom I meet as a client, on the street, or connect with throughout the pages of this book. You need to know and remember we all have purpose in Christ; we all have reason for being here on earth. Life is a journey to walk out this truth, and I want to help optimize this.

So, it starts here— building a foundation of greatness through true health and wellness, a foundation that is faith-based and empowers you to be your best whole self, so you can give your best to those who need it. This is what it's all about and what Christ focused on daily. Personally, I feel most alive when I am giving, helping, or tending to someone in need.

> Acts 20:35 AMP, *"In everything I showed you [by example] that by working hard in this way you must help the weak and remember the words of the Lord Jesus, that He Himself said, 'It is more blessed [and brings greater joy] to give than to receive.'"*

I may not always feel like it, but I know it is better to give than receive. Think about the last time you reached out to help someone in need. How did it feel? Selfless giving is a gift in and of itself. Part of these pages will help you get to a place where you can come from this spiritual place of giving, the way scripture has called you to live and love.

My focus in all of this centers around two principles: *prevention* and *consistency*. Preventing the things the world brings, such as pain, sickness, disease, obesity, depression, anxiety, and so on. With less of this in your life you can begin to come from a place of consistent outreach to those in need. *You can begin to look forward and not down.*

Yet, I know and understand this is not the way the world works, and sometimes, it can even seem like everything is against this kind of living (which I believe it is). *I want you to know that you were built for consistency.* Consistently loving, living, praying, and walking in the Spirit, this is the goal, and I have a strong conviction to help you rise to the calling.

I did not, however, start my wellness journey with this conviction. In 2014, I had an idea for a company I call 360wellness. I began this health and wellness startup with a simple Instagram profile focused on corrective exercise, nutrition, and prevention while simultaneously discovering my passions junior year of college. As I continued into my senior year, I gained experience in the healthcare industry working under amazing physical therapists as a physical therapy aide (someone who assists the physical therapist in rehab-based procedures and exercises).

Through my work, I connected with two amazing therapists, Nadar and Mary, who were both Christian and had come from Egypt looking to start a life in America. Over many years, they developed a successful physical therapy business named Agape Physical Therapy (agape happens to mean unconditional love; God's love).

I will not forget the day I applied for an internship at Agape.

As I was driving by and hesitant to apply for an internship position, something pulled on my heart (which I later learned was a nudge from the Holy Spirit). I ended up pulling a U-turn and going inside. This ultimately led me to work with them for an entire year while I finished my degree at Azusa Pacific University in Southern California. I learned amazing concepts and applications in the rehab field that I still use with clients today. However, I felt there was something missing in this kind of care, and I was hungry to bridge the gap.

While I was involved in my internship, I learned two things:

The first is that I was empathetic toward my clients, and it broke my heart. Every time I would work with someone in pain from post-surgery or an injury, I wished there had been a way to prevent it. It seemed like 80% of the cases coming through could have been prevented if caught early. The second is that the healthcare system unfortunately made it difficult for the patient and the provider to do what they needed to do for full recovery (along with prevention of further pain/injury). There just wasn't enough time or money to solve the issue at hand.

As I graduated, I continued my journey and found my true relationship with God. After moving to San Diego, I realized He was leading me on a unique path. *I recognized the power of faith in Jesus Christ and the healing, health, and peace that comes with it.* I call this kind of peace "true peace." There are many things available to us that provide a temporary peace, but through faith and relationship with God, there's an opportunity for something deeper, something that is true and lasting. Jesus is the missing piece in wellness that very few professionals can and are emphasizing in their model of client care. I want things to change. *This application to your life satisfies and allows you to graduate to a place of Godly leadership and love, founding characteristics of greatness.*

This view has led me to continually evolve 360wellness, as the concepts have with it. I always had a foundation of preventative health and well-being in the beginning, with massage, exercise, nutrition, and mindfulness being the founding concepts. I quickly learned what my fitness and therapy clients needed most for a balanced life. As time went on, God began to lead me toward the Christ-centered focus on health. Christ is our cornerstone, and without Him, we have nothing.

> John 15:5 *"I am the Vine; you are the branches. The one who remains in Me and I in him bears much fruit, for [otherwise] apart from Me [that is, cut off from vital union with Me] you can do nothing."*

My vision began to change. My passions began to change.

God began to transform 360wellness. Over time, it has become the way I know He intended it to be. It impacts others past the physical level, empowering the Body of Christ to be who they were created to be. This vision became clearer at the end of 2019, when I received a word from God saying, *"We Will See*

Clearly. " As I write in the middle of the year 2020, I can begin to see that eyes are opening to what should be truly valued in life and the gift of life that oftentimes we forget to be grateful for.

It is time for change. One may say a pivot. I therefore believe in proclaiming a health that doesn't just focus on the physical and mental aspects of a person, but also supports the spirit with a Christ-centered mindset. *This is wholeness. This is where everything flows. You do not have complete health without the spirit being nurtured and tended to.*

My passion and calling is to bridge the gap between healthcare and the Church: providing support, direction, and training for the body of Christ, helping to maximize its impact. Imagine a holistic healthcare system open to God's love and Spirit, freely and openly confessing that Christ is Lord while providing elite professional care to all who will come.

This would be a place where prayer is a part of culture and the healing process. A place where you have faith-based care from working professionals who want to see you live your best life for God's glory. This has been building inside of me, and I have a dream to one day make a global impact with 360wellness through a system capable of helping others find health and wholeness across the globe. This would cultivate a culture of helping to empower churches, third-world communities, the less-fortunate in America, the homeless, and the broken.

Does this sound like a lot? Let me begin with the foundation. I realize the importance and power in integrating the holistic health of the body, mind, and spirit. I also know your potential. This way of living will maximize and give clarity to your walk of faith in our complex efforts to become whole. I look at wholeness as a state of working toward health in not just the body, but also the mind and spirit. I believe it is a continual process and is a precursor to what I call "true wellness."

As you work toward this foundation, you are able to set up God (and the Holy Spirit) to be most active in your life— seeing clearly, walking in purity (of all kinds), and limiting the distractions of this world. However, in addition to God's grace, you will have to take diligent, intentional, organized action. For faith without works is dead (James 2:26). Within the Body of Christ, there is a need to become more proactive with our holistic health: to live with prevention in mind.

To be proactive is defined as, *"(of a person or action) creating or controlling a situation by causing something to happen rather than responding to it after it has happened"* (Oxford Dictionaries, 2020).

On paper, maintaining this kind of holistic health is easy. Stay active, eat your veggies, build long-lasting support and connection with others, consistently pray, read scripture, and so on. If you are being realistic, however, things— kids, injury, pain, lack of motivation, distractions, and other priorities (or idols) — get in the way. Before we walk through the concepts of my philosophy on wholeness, I would like to call out and identify some of the reasons and/or *lies* that might keep you from building a foundation of true wellness in your life.

1. Knowledge

You might not be truly aware of the benefits of self-care, exercise, sound nutrition, sleep, stress management, prayer, and the practices alike. Knowledge AND action are power.

2. Support

It's hard to do it alone and that's ok. That's normal. All of us need support, direction, and encouragement throughout life. The same applies to your health. I believe everyone should have a coach or mentor to help maximize their potential.

Seek those around you whom you can trust. Tell them your story and your goals. You never know, they may even be motivated and want to start a connect group.

3. *"It's vanity"*

During this day and age, the fitness industry sexualizes health. Many people want to look better to impress others, gaining a kind of confidence and self-worth from body image. That isn't what this book is about. I'd like to say there are always two ways of doing things. They both may look the same, but it's all about intention. Where the heart is matters (Matthew 15:18).

Health is much deeper than the physical. And the good thing about it? The outside always reflects the care you do on the inside. *The more you care for your body with pure intentions, the more you'll notice the true "you" starting to show.*

This has always reminded me of Jesus preaching, *"seek first the kingdom of God"* (Matthew 6:33). First tend to yourself from the inside-out with righteousness. All you are looking for will come from that place. There's no need to strive.

We all have a certain body type— the way God made us. The more you change your mindset from how the world views health and fitness, the more you can be realistic and content with your body, tending to yourself as a temple of God, not something to disgrace.

4. *"I'm not good enough/worth it"*

This is a lie. The devil is a liar, and the fact that you are alive and breathing today shows you have purpose; you may just need to find it. If you think no one else believes in you, I do. I trust you are on to great things for the sake of others if you allow yourself to believe.

Yet, you must know that consistency in life starts with self-care. If you pour into others without pouring into yourself, how can you be your best? How can you give your best? Perspective is everything. And You. Are. Worth. It.

Believe me; it's not always about how you feel. *Sometimes you just have to walk by faith and watch it grow.* You must see everyone's potential reflected in the image of God. This is where unconditional love begins— a love for God, self, and others because first and foremost you were made in His image. You are a Son or Daughter. Your potential is everything, and Jesus was sent to restore that. *Do you not know who you are?*

5. *"I don't have time"*

This may feel true. We all experience overwhelming pressure from work, responsibility, daily tasks, family, and personal goals, but it's always a matter of priority. Time will always be limited, and it cannot be renewed. *You have to decide to make the time, no matter how small it may be.* Even just a few minutes daily, or 10% effort, can yield huge results in the long run. To maximize your potential, it's all about prioritizing and staying consistent. Find your marathon pace!

6. *"It's just not my thing"*

That's fair. Taking weekly spa days, working out in the gym 7 days a week, becoming an ordained minister, and prepping organic cooked meals with your personal chef may not be realistic. You may not even have an interest. And that's ok. *There is no perfect route or process here.* You just need to find what you enjoy and be realistic. You can do your best with what God has given you. The beautiful thing is God meets you where you are at, giving you more to manage when you can handle it.

> Matthew 25:29, *"For to everyone who has [and values his blessings and gifts from God, and has used them wisely], more will be given, and [he will be richly supplied so that] he will have an abundance; but from the one who does not have [because he has ignored or disregarded his blessings and gifts from God], even what he does have will be taken away."*

7. *Filling a void*

Lastly, you may use certain lifestyle habits (fast food, social media, alcohol, caffeine) as a filler, but let me encourage and remind you, only God will satisfy and sustain your insatiable need for love, wholeness, and peace. *He is with you and you are not alone in this.* If you can have faith to break through the fog, even for a few seconds, building healthy habits and finding support (in the body, mind, and spirit) can provide the fulfillment you truly seek.

No matter what, the foundation of health stays the same. Focus on your health and understand it because you matter, you will be your best, and you will feel your best throughout this journey of life. No matter what trials the world brings, or what opportunities you have to pour into others, you will be making an impact in people's lives and in God's kingdom wherever He plants you. So, don't believe the lies.

This book is a philosophy on wholeness, a philosophy on how you can heal from and prevent the world's negative impact on the body, mind, and spirit. It's also a solution to help you optimize your wellness and maximize your God-given potential so you can walk as an influencer in this world. As a lion, not a sheep, for the glory of God.

In the next 7 chapters, I have created a healthy, integrated foundation of wholeness for the body, mind, and spirit. *God wants you to shine, and I call out the gold in you.* Everyone's greatness may look different, but it's up to you and your perspective to make the most of what you have in this world and aim to be your best. This is a race. Your life matters. *You were created for greatness.*

1 Corinthians 9:24-27 AMP, *"Do you not know that in a race all the runners run [their very best to win], but only one receives the prize? Run [your race] in such a way that you may seize the prize and make it yours! Now every athlete who [goes into training and] competes in the games is disciplined and exercises self-control in all things. They do it to win a crown that withers, but we [do it to receive] an imperishable [crown that cannot wither].*

Therefore I do not run without a definite goal; I do not flail around like one beating the air [just shadow boxing]. But [like a boxer] I strictly discipline my body and make it my slave, so that, after I have preached [the gospel] to others, I myself will not somehow be disqualified [as unfit for service]."

Reflect

Consider the 7 reasons/lies that might be keeping you from building a true foundation of wellness in your life. Which one do you find yourself thinking about most often? How would your life look differently if you were free from that belief/obstacle?

Chapter I – The Concept

1 Timothy 4:8 AMP, *"For physical training is of some value, but godliness (spiritual training) is of value in everything and in every way, since it holds promise for the present life and for the life to come."*

In a world of pain, sickness, and disease, something needs to change. You can no longer go on just getting by. There must be action. There must be change. You must become serious about your wellness so you can consistently accomplish all that God intends for your life.

Wellness is not limited to just your physical body; it expands into your mental, emotional, and spiritual self. This can best be explained through the biopsychosocial model, which considers multiple aspects of your life as keys to wellness. These include biological (such as age), psychological (such as mental health), and sociological (such as environment or social support) factors. I would also add spiritual health to this list, but more on that later.

Time and time again, people fall to pain, addiction, depression, lack of motivation, and purpose, yet we are called to greatness. Whatever this looks like to you, as a Believer, you should come from a place of abundance and rest to help those in need along your path. You are truly called to give.

Acts 20:35 AMP, *"In everything I showed you [by example] that by working hard in this way you must help the weak and remember the words of the Lord Jesus, that He Himself said, 'It is more blessed [and brings greater joy] to give than to receive.'"*

But how can you truly give without first becoming whole yourself? From a foundational, personal point of view, you need to empower others to become whole, so that as the Church (body of Christ), we can reach out with selfless love to those in need. The following examples are related to the *flesh*, or human nature, and can leave you in a box focused on *self*, whether you realize it or not. I call them "distractions."

- Pain

- Sickness

- Disease

- Depression

- Anxiety

- Fear

- Obesity

I'd like to touch on obesity. I am not by any means talking about those who are naturally larger than the status quo of "fit." *God has made all of mankind with different shapes, sizes, and metabolisms, so don't let anyone tell you otherwise. That is a lie from the pit of hell, and I bind and rebuke in the name of Jesus Christ any insecurity or self-doubt regarding body image to those reading this page. God loves you so much.* If you are struggling with your weight, don't agree with anything else.

What I am referring to when I say obesity is when you overeat and begin to weigh beyond your natural weight. This lifestyle can not only become harmful to your physiological body (heart, hormone, and mental health) but also to your spiritual health, as it deals with feeding the "flesh" and can lead to other distractions mentioned above. You need to be incredibly careful of the fine line between enjoying your freedom and gluttony, which is rarely discussed in the Church. I will discuss this further in chapter 4.

So, these seven distractions may be "normal," but as a child of God, you are not called to these things. *As part of the body of Christ, you are called to health, life, and dominion, using these things to focus on others, dying to self, and picking up your cross daily to follow Jesus.* It seems almost contradicting, yet it is a truly balanced way of life.

> Genesis 1:26 AMP, *"Then God said, 'Let Us (Father, Son, Holy Spirit) make man in Our image, according to Our likeness [not physical, but a spiritual personality and moral likeness]; and let them have complete authority over the fish of the sea, the birds of the air, the cattle, and over the entire earth, and over everything that creeps and crawls on the earth.'"*

> Luke 9:23 AMP, *"And He was saying to them all, 'If anyone wishes to follow Me [as My disciple], he must deny himself [set aside selfish interests], and take up his cross daily [expressing a willingness to endure whatever may come] and follow Me [believing in Me, conforming to My example in living and, if need be, suffering or perhaps dying because of faith in Me].'"*

> Luke 4:18 NASB, *"THE SPIRIT OF THE LORD IS UPON ME (the Messiah), because He has anointed Me to preach the good news to the poor. He has sent Me to announce release (pardon, forgiveness) TO THE CAPTIVES, and recovery of sight to the blind, to set free those who are oppressed (downtrodden, bruised, crushed by tragedy)."*

Jesus sets free those who are oppressed. You're not called to sit in your room and be "Godly." You're called to go out into the world and make an impact (Matthew 28:29). The journey will not be easy but who ever said it would be, or should be? *The influence of this world is doing everything in its power to stop your true greatness from manifesting.* The flesh, the world, and the devil, with all of their confusion, distractions, and temptations, are in direct opposition to what we are called to walk in– the Spirit (Galatians 5). You must be alert and do everything in your best interest for the kingdom of God (which is righteousness, peace, and joy).

> Romans 14:17 NASB, *"For the kingdom of God is not eating and drinking, but righteousness and peace and joy in the Holy Spirit."*

What you need to realize is that this life is not about you and never has been. Serve God. Serve others. In this, you will find true freedom and joy, taking the focus off yourself.

> Galatians 5:13 AMP, *"For you, my brothers, were called to freedom; only do not let your freedom become an opportunity for the sinful nature (worldliness, selfishness), but through love serve and seek the best for one another."*

> John 8:31-32 AMP, *"So Jesus was saying to the Jews who had believed Him, 'If you abide in My word [continually obeying My teachings and living in accordance with them, then] you are truly My disciples. And you will know the truth [regarding salvation], and the truth will set you free [from the penalty of sin].'"*

> Matthew 10:39 AMP, *"Whoever finds his life [in this world] will [eventually] lose it [through death], and whoever loses his life [in this world] for My sake will find it [that is, life with Me for all eternity]."*

Yet, we still must value ourselves as the temple of God and obey God's word.

> 1 Corinthians 3:16 AMP, *"Do you not know and understand that you [the church] are the temple of God, and that the Spirit of God dwells [permanently] in you [collectively and individually]?"*

> 2 Corinthians 6:16 AMP, *"What agreement is there between the temple of God and idols? For we are the temple of the living God; just as God said: 'I WILL DWELL IN THEM AND WALK AMONG THEM; AND I WILL BE THEIR GOD, AND THEY SHALL BE MY PEOPLE.'"*

The following pages will explain and walk you through each concept of wellness to promote wholeness. This is what I believe makes up a solid foundation for your walk as a Believer. I am with you throughout this journey and only have your best interests in mind. What I believe God has spoken directly to my heart is to, "Heal My People." I know He is talking about you. The Church. God's people. His chosen.

There is brokenness and hurt in the body of Christ, but I call for restoration. Not for personal gain, as I am not doing this for money or attention, but solely from the heart, through what God has taught me on my own journey (and is continuing to teach me). It has been 6 years since the first vision of 360wellness, and it continues to evolve as God leads this fluid company.

I have come to realize the Gospel is a holistic message, and I must integrate this into what I do. I believe with all my heart that the body affects the mind/spirit and vice versa, yet rarely do we apply intention to this. This mentality has brought me to start a business that focuses on the preventative health of God's people and all who will come.

At the end of the day, my foundation in all of this is prevention and consistency. In this day and age, being prevention-focused and consistent with your actions is essential. You must begin to act against your sedentary jobs, quick result mindsets ("microwave mentality"), lust of food and drink, high stress environments, self-centeredness, and the distractions of pain, sickness, and disease that the world so easily creates for you.

I continue to call these things distractions because they can pull us away from our number one purpose: to consistently love God and others.

> Matthew 22:36-39 AMP, *"'Teacher, which is the greatest commandment in the Law?' And Jesus replied to him, 'YOU SHALL LOVE THE LORD YOUR GOD WITH ALL YOUR HEART, AND WITH ALL YOUR SOUL, AND WITH ALL YOUR MIND.' This is the first and greatest commandment. The second is like it, 'YOU SHALL LOVE YOUR NEIGHBOR AS YOURSELF [that is, unselfishly seek the best or higher good for others].'"*

It's hard to help or pray for someone else when you are distracted and dealing with your own "issues." Do you have to be perfect and have everything figured out? Of course not. But you aren't called to this kind of life.

Yes, as humans we have in a way brought this upon ourselves. The environment we grew up in, our busy lives, incredible demands at work, and the food and drink industries are just giving us what we want, but there's the problem— it's *what we want*. But it's not entirely your fault. In some ways, you've been born into it. From the type of family you grew up with, to the fast-paced culture you live in today, you learned to adopt certain habits and mindsets.

Personally, I was raised in Texas. My family was small, simple, and taught to finish the food left on the plate. To enjoy Bluebell ice cream every chance you had, and if you were old enough (or not) to have a beer and "loosen up". *Self-control and health were a second thought. This was culture. This is culture.*

Your lifestyle may look different to you now than it did in your past, but the foundations of this worldly culture are the same, and unfortunately, they do not produce good, lasting fruit. They are not centered in Christ. Through my own experience and working with clients of every background, there is a better way. *You can no longer carry these habits or related ones with you into a maturing Christian life.*

Notice I say maturing. As a Christian, you are called to more by regarding our body as God's temple now that we host the Holy Spirit (1 Corinthians 3:16-17). Another scripture that has been a foundation for my life and 360wellness (yet isn't discussed often in healthcare or the Church) is 1 Timothy 4:8 (AMP),

> *"For physical training is of some value, but godliness (spiritual training) is of value in everything and in every way, since it holds promise for the present life and for the life to come."*

This book is not just about taking action and caring for your physical and mental state. It's also about taking care of your spirit and integrating the action of faith into your walk as a Believer. Most of the concepts throughout the following pages, you will know. They may be taken to a new depth, but they are used by most of us. There's one, however, that seems less common. It is the integration of health and wellness into the Christian Body— a place where science freely meets Faith.

In the technology and progress of today, you must be proactive in healthcare, wellness, and new applications within the Church, and that's ok. As the distractions (of the world) and accessibility to those distractions rise, your actions must go "from glory to glory" in all areas of life.

> 2 Corinthians 3:17-18 AMP, *"Now the Lord is the Spirit, and where the Spirit of the Lord is, there is liberty [emancipation from bondage, true freedom]. And we all, with unveiled face, continually seeing as in a mirror the glory of the Lord, are progressively being transformed into His image from [one degree of] glory to [even more] glory, which comes from the Lord, [who is] the Spirit."*

You must begin to think and act differently to be set apart from the ways of the world. As you are continually transformed into the image of Christ, your day-to-day actions need to transform with you all the way down to healthy, foundational wellness. We're talking "the mind of Christ." This is stewarding well all that God has given you. Imagine if the Christian Church lived with this conviction: *That you are enough and that YOU can have the impact God desires in your life through tending to your wellness.* True wellness consistently, not just in the body but also in mind and spirit.

You must move past the "old-school" way of doing things, acting by sheer will, even shaming others (or yourself) for not keeping up or staying consistent. You need direction and new application to walk consistently in purity of the body, mind, and spirit as a Believer. The worldly influence around you does not make it easy, so this holistic kind of thinking is what, I believe, true wellness boils down to.

> Matthew 26:40-41 AMP, *"And He came to the disciples and found them sleeping, and said to Peter, 'So,*

you men could not stay awake and keep watch with Me
for one hour? Keep actively watching and praying that
you may not come into temptation; the spirit is willing,
but the body is weak.'"

You can no longer continue off willpower and good intentions if you want to maximize your impact, lead as a good example, and empower the lives of others as Christ commanded. As a Believer you have the Holy Spirit, but you have to set up the Holy Spirit to be used in your life. You must not limit the power of God. You must not limit the Holy One of Israel. There is a choice. There's always a choice. God always looks for someone to rise to the occasion but finds few.

Matthew 22:14 AMP, *"For many are called (invited, summoned), but few are chosen."*

You become available for more opportunity by creating a temple dedicated to hosting the Lord's Spirit and living a life of purity in all areas of your life (limiting the flesh and not squandering our freedom/power, Galatians 5:13). This is foundational and essential to the Christian Body for full potential.

I know from reading scripture that spiritual warfare is happening all around us. The last thing the devil wants is for you to walk dressed in the identity God has given you. I also know the flesh (sinful nature) and the world (unrighteous culture) are at war against your potential. You must level up as a Believer and take action in what you can control. God doesn't want you to be immature. He wants Godly men and women who will learn, grow, and take responsibility in caring for His living temple (our body). The Bible calls this stewardship. *Don't miss this: not by satisfying your desires, but by being good stewards of what God has given you.*

It's actually an act of worship to care for what God has created.

1 Corinthians 3:1-3 AMP, *"However, brothers and sisters, I could not talk to you as to spiritual people, but [only] as to worldly people [dominated by human nature], mere infants [in the new life] in Christ! I fed you with milk, not solid food; for you were not yet able to receive it. Even now you are still not ready. You are still worldly [controlled by ordinary impulses, the sinful capacity]. For as long as there is jealousy and strife and discord among you, are you not unspiritual, and are you not walking like ordinary men [unchanged by faith]?"*

Romans 12:1 AMP, *"Therefore I urge you, brothers and sisters, by the mercies of God, to present your bodies [dedicating all of yourselves, set apart] as a living sacrifice, holy and well-pleasing to God, which is your rational (logical, intelligent) act of worship."*

No longer should you, or can you, go on giving into the lusts of the world. Overindulging in social media and food, while sexualized fitness, easy access to drinking/drugs, "busyness," self-centeredness, and the stress of performance stand in your way. They pull you away from who you truly are called to be, what you were created for: *Greatness.* Because of this, it is necessary you learn to plan, prioritize, and build healthy habits. Thus, taking intentional action in all areas of your life to stay consistent in your health and walk with God.

Romans 8:10-11 AMP, *"If Christ lives in you, though your [natural] body is dead because of sin, your spirit is alive because of righteousness [which He provides]. And if the Spirit of Him who raised Jesus from the dead lives in you, He who raised Christ Jesus from the dead will also give life to your mortal bodies through His Spirit, who lives in you."*

As you are a balance of the body and the soul, my philosophy is a balance of the practical and spiritual. The Holy Spirit, who quickens your own, is just as much a part of your wellness as the mind and body, actually allowing you the self-control and mind of Christ needed to walk consistently in this way of life (not by how much we strive to change).

> John 16:7 AMP, *"But I tell you the truth, it is your advantage that I go away; for if I do not go away, the helper (comforter, advocate, intercessor – counselor, strengthener, standby) will not come to you; but if I go, I will send Him (the Holy Spirit) to you [to be in close fellowship with you]."*

To put it plainly, you are changed from the inside out by your time spent with the Lord, His presence, and receiving it daily (2 Corinthians 3:17). I refer to this as true rest, or what some call "devotional rest." It's one of the most difficult things you will obtain. Damon Thompson, a worldwide revivalist, says it this way, *"the most difficult thing you'll say yes to in your life, is an end to personal, devotional inconsistency."* This is where prioritizing organization, faith, and spiritual strength come in (we'll dive deeper into this concept in chapter 7).

Finally, I present you with the keys of wellness that make up the foundation of 360wellness: *Recovery, Exercise, Nutrition, Mindfulness, and Faith.* In each chapter of this book, you will learn more about the individual keys, and by exploring these five concepts through a biblical lens, I trust you can and will live a fulfilled life through every mountain and valley. You will be ready to love others with a content and purpose-driven heart, the way God intended for all of us.

Living with greatness.

<u>The 5 Whys:</u> as you move forward, this coaching exercise will help your process. It will also help you remember the deeper, personal meaning of this book and how it relates to you. Take your time, answering each *why*, starting with your reason for reading *You Were Created For Greatness*.

The following *whys* will begin to break down the true root of your purpose. May God bless you and guide you.

1. Why are you reading this book?

2. Awesome. Why?

3. Ok, and why is this important to you?

4. Why?

5. Lastly, Why?

Thank you. This is your root, or core belief and purpose behind choosing to read this book.

Reflect

Use the space below to complete The 5 Whys exercise.

Chapter II – Recovery

Psalm 23:1-3 AMP, *"The LORD is my Shepherd [to feed, to guide and to shield me], I shall not want. He lets me lie down in green pastures; He leads me beside the still and quiet waters. He refreshes and restores my soul (life); He leads me in the paths of righteousness for His name's sake."*

You must care for yourself to care well for others. Ask yourself, *"Do I give enough to myself, to give my best to others?"* This holds true in all areas of life. You can't give what you don't have (for long). So, if the answer is "no" – this book is for you. There's a fine line between powering through a pain or injury and humbling yourself to receive help. I've seen God use an injury many times to teach and slow people down (including myself).

Before I start with any client looking to improve their rehab, health, fitness, diet, and/or lifestyle habits, I encourage holistic *recovery* as a priority. Most of the time, 9 out of 10 people deal with some type of pain, injury (current or past), lack of sleep, and stress or tightness in their body (or mind) that can create, what I call, an imbalance. We all deal with things daily that pull us away from being in a balanced state.

In order to stay consistent and come from a place of abundance, you must have this internal, holistic balance from the inside out. To acknowledge this and then act on that awareness is foundational to well-being. Literally.

Please acknowledge this. You must take time to recover and balance yourself if you are going to stay consistent in your walk for the long haul. I find the benefits of this include, but are not limited to, minimizing distractions, maximizing potential, enjoying the process, and preventing burnout wherever God calls you. You may just need to *rest*. Particularly if you're reading this coming out of 2020, your body has been in a chronic state of stress and isolation which can cause more than one health-problem. In a world of striving and progress, you need to slow down within the storms.

> Have you read Zechariah 4:6 AMP? *"Then he said to me, 'This [continuous supply of oil] is the word of the* LORD *to Zerubbabel [prince of Judah], saying, 'Not by might, nor by power, but by My Spirit [of whom the oil is a symbol],' says the* LORD *of hosts.'"*

As humans, we tend to choose *striving* over *striding*, yet, as a Believer you now have someone who fights on your behalf and can give you the strength you need in any weakness (2 Chronicles 32:7-8, 2 Corinthians 12:10, Romans 8:26). The idea is to abide. *This is the final piece: rest for your spirit, which adds rest to your mind, body, and soul.*

Through experience with a wide range of clients, I have found that whether you are active or sedentary, you must take the time to balance and recover yourself through intentional rest. The human body is adaptive and smart, yet fragile. It can adjust to your workload, posture, hobbies, lifestyle, and daily habits but sooner or later imbalances begin to show. It is only a matter of time. This is usually in the form of burnout, pain, injury, and/or "tightness" in the body (surprisingly, tightness has been found to be a neurological affect more than a tight "knot" as society once believed).

Think of a car. The faster you go, the more pressure is put on the engine, shocks, and tires. If the car is not aligned (e.g., imbalances, low-tire pressure, dirty oil), you will experience wear and tear, not to mention low performance. In some cases, it may even begin to fall apart. However, *You Were Made to Move.*

This is one *360 Mindset* I have based my business on. To take it one step further: *you were made to move, well!* I want to see you progress and live a joyful, balanced, pain-free life, and it starts with a foundation of recovery.

Below are 5 practical ways to integrate more of it into your life today:

1. Relax, take a walk

Sometimes it can be simple. Taking the time to slow down and take a 5-minute walk has been shown to do wonders for stress management and boosting muscle recovery. Lowering stress levels can calm the nervous system (in turn lowering cortisol) and cause us to "reset" in the middle of the day, at the end of a stressful shift, or even as we get the day started off right.

Fun fact, the release of cortisol is a normal and helpful anti-inflammatory response, but if released chronically, it can lead to health issues such as weight gain and increased inflammation. It can even lower your immune system response!

2. Targeted therapy

360wellness was founded on combining targeted massage with active stretching. The keyword here is *targeted.* By localizing the area of tension and pain, we can recover the body faster and add efficiency to your recovery routine. If possible, especially when dealing with pain or injury, search for a therapist in your area who focuses on acute, therapeutic massage. It's ok, you deserve it.

Are you not into massage? Is it not in your budget? No worries, I can relate. I bring you another option and a great tool (not a solution) — foam rollers. A foam roller releases muscle tension by improving blood flow. You can lay on it, press against the wall, or use it in a seated chair position. This release is temporary, as the body will usually go back to its "comfortable" position (posture is commonly formed through repetitive movements), but it's a great start and has become a part of many athletes' recovery routine.

3. Breathe deep

Just five deep breaths a day can be a great start in reducing stress, lowering your heart rate and blood pressure, all while decreasing your cortisol levels. I recommend setting a timer on your phone when you know your day is at its busiest to help break the cycle of stress. You can take this small, daily action and put it to use for a surprising boost to your wellness.

Try this: "Box Breathing" is an awesome tool to slow down, breathe deep, and maximize oxygen. Start by inhaling for 5 seconds (through your nose), then hold for 5 seconds, exhale for 5 seconds (through your mouth), and hold for 5 seconds, then repeat. It takes a little bit of getting used to, but only one round can be just what you need to reset during the day!

4. Movement is medicine

Not many people think of movement itself as recovery. I am thankful for many great mentors in my life, showing me the way. One of them, Dominick Nusdeu of Motion

Mechanix, showed me the value of movement as a substitute to massage therapy. Yes, replacing massage with movement. As I'm a licensed massage therapist, we had our brotherly disagreements, but he pointed me to a view of how the body functions that I hadn't seen before. His concept was to create stability in certain ranges of motion. This is meant to challenge your mobility and find strength in an array of different movements (what he calls "configurations"). When these range of motion exercises are applied over time, most tightness, pain, and lack of stability in joints disappear. It's pretty amazing, and I have now fused it with my targeted massage program to accelerate the healing process.

The basic principle is this: you must stabilize the specific joint of pain/tightness with movement. If your shoulder is experiencing tightness, stabilize it. If your knee is experiencing pain, stabilize it. And so on. Time and time again, I've seen pain, tension, and "tightness" all be caused by instability of the joint (which happens to also affect your posture and strength). If you start with small movements to improve posture and the connection of the focused area, the relief will amaze you. I could write all day about this, but I'll leave you with one last tip: If you move a certain direction and there is pain/discomfort, stop and try the same movement but in the opposite direction (and hold).

For example, if your knee bothers you when bending, straighten it out and hold for 5-10 seconds (like a knee extension exercise). If your low back hurts when bending over, lay down and extend your body back with a bridge exercise. If your neck feels tight when turning to the left, slowly turn to the right and hold. This technique will begin to stabilize (or balance) the body's "push-pull" relationship. Whether you are new to exercise or a seasoned expert, you can begin to apply this technique today for a great start to recovery.

Here's what it could look like if you organized these into your warm-up routine:

1. *Seated Knee Extensions - 2 sets of 3 reps (10 second hold)*
2. *Bridges -2 sets of 3 reps (10 second hold)*
3. *Neck Rotation - 2 sets of 3 reps each way (10 second hold)*

5. Rest

Maybe the MOST important factor of recovery is sleep. Research has shown sleep is the most powerful recovery technique we can give to ourselves, and it's free! Praise the Lord. Between 7-9 hours is a healthy range, however, just as important of a factor is sleep *quality*. This is a personal goal of mine (something that I must stay mindful of daily) and another *360 Mindset* I live by: *Quality Over Quantity.* You can sleep for hours, but if it's not quality, deep sleep, you may not get the full recovery benefits.

So, here are a few restful ideas to implement into your growing holistic lifestyle, thanks to **Precision Nutrition**, a world-renowned nutrition and lifestyle-coaching program. While just a few ideas are provided, I encourage you to highlight those that relate to you. Then choose *ONE* to focus on and apply for 1-2 weeks until you have built a habit.

Here are my top 6 ideas:

- Stick to a routine bedtime (the mind and body like consistent timing)

- Turn off electronics at least 30 minutes before bed (screen time can reduce sleep quality)
- Journal (write out your thoughts, ideas, and/or emotions to help ease your mind)
- Keep your room dark (add blackout curtains or try a sleep mask to promote deep, REM sleep)
- Exercise regularly (aim for 20-60 minutes daily as this promotes restful sleep and helps manage energy)
- Apply a 5-minute prayer time to your bed-time routine (spend time with God and rest in the "secret place")

Psalm 91 (NIV): one of my favorite passages to read out loud and *rest* (meditate) in before bed is a song of King David who had a deep, personal relationship with God. We will dive deeper into this specific kind of rest in chapter 7.

¹ Whoever dwells in the shelter of the Most High
will rest in the shadow of the Almighty.

² I will say of the LORD, "He is my refuge and my fortress,
my God, in whom I trust."

³ Surely he will save you
from the fowler's snare
and from the deadly pestilence.

⁴ He will cover you with his feathers,
and under his wings you will find refuge;
His faithfulness will be your shield and rampart.

⁵ You will not fear the terror of night,
nor the arrow that flies by day,

⁶ nor the pestilence that stalks in the darkness,
   nor the plague that destroys at midday.

⁷ A thousand may fall at your side,
   ten thousand at your right hand,
   but it will not come near you.

⁸ You will only observe with your eyes
   and see the punishment of the wicked.

⁹ If you say, "The LORD is my refuge,"
and you make the Most High your dwelling,

¹⁰ no harm will overtake you,
   no disaster will come near your tent.

¹¹ For he will command his angels concerning you
   to guard you in all your ways;

¹² they will lift you up in their hands,
so that you will not strike your foot against a stone.

¹³ You will tread on the lion and the cobra;
   you will trample the great lion and the serpent.

¹⁴ "Because he loves me," says the LORD, "I will rescue him;
I will protect him, for he acknowledges my name.

¹⁵ He will call on me, and I will answer him;
   I will be with him in trouble,
   I will deliver him and honor him.

¹⁶ With long life I will satisfy him
   and show him my salvation."

In the next chapter, you will learn about my concept of exercise and how you can use simple actions to help improve your life for the better. *But first, as a Believer, you must differentiate the Church and your mentality from the way the world sees fitness and health.*

Reflect

Do you give enough to yourself so that you can give your best to others? Consider the 5 practical ways to integrate recovery into your life. What do you want to start incorporating this week? How will you accomplish this?

Chapter III – Exercise

Romans 12:2 AMP, *"And do not be conformed to this world [any longer with its superficial values and customs], but be transformed and progressively changed [as you mature spiritually] by the renewing of your mind [focusing on godly values and ethical attitudes], so that you may prove [for yourselves] what the will of God is, that which is good and acceptable and perfect [in His plan and purpose for you]."*

Growing up, exercise was simple. For me as a kid, it involved tag, hide and go seek, dodgeball, you name it. It was easy, and it was fun. There were no strings attached, and there was no real pressure to look or be a certain way.

As we grow up, however, the idea of exercise begins to take a shift. Things change. Unfortunately, most of what movies, commercials, trainers, social media, and gyms promote is a sexualized fitness. This way of living is not sustainable or healthy for many reasons. Many of you are tempted to aim for unrealistic goals, setting you up for lies and disappointment.

Instead, let us focus on this: God loves you no matter your size, shape, color, or how "different" you may feel. *There is a deeper meaning and purpose to life than to satisfy the physical need or image the world reflects.* Everyone else may be doing it, even striving for it, yet you are called to stand out from the crowd and not give in. You are called to go so far as to continually transform your mind, leading as new examples to others. I'm talking about being counterintuitive.

It is important for the church to understand that exercise focused on our image will not produce the good fruit or freedom we desire. As small as it may be, the enemy can use this foothold in your life to plant lies and distract you from your true identity. This understanding is especially essential as the fitness industry only continues to expand and sexualize this kind of image-based fitness.

So, I call you back to the basics. Exercise, no matter what it looks like, is important for a healthy life. Let's review the definition.

According to Oxford Dictionary, exercise is *"a process or activity carried out for a specific purpose, especially one concerned with a specified area or skill."*

I love this definition because no matter the specifics, *you* are taking action for a purpose. Some may define this as being intentional. Consistent health is all about intention, and I genuinely believe as humans, we were made to move. The body is capable of more than you challenge it with, and I encourage you to explore that potential. Along with this, there are hundreds of benefits to exercise.

Here are just a few that stand out to me:

1. Improves your circulation
2. Increases your bone density
3. Regulates your mood
4. Challenges your comfort-zone (supports mental resilience)
5. Supports a healthy metabolism

The more you stay moving, the better chance you have at living a robust, happy, long, healthy life. With factors ranging from stress-relief, weight control, and pain management, I have seen movement improve quality of life from the young to the old. *360 Mindset - Movement is Medicine.*

As I work with many clients dealing with pain, I can see the healing benefits of movement. Again, it may seem counterintuitive, but staying active is the one thing that outshines other rehabilitation and prevention techniques. It is *effective* and *free*. All you have to do is start moving, with *intention*.

Think of a child in development: moldable, eager, and willing to try new things. No matter what type of exercise you prefer, I encourage you to keep this simplicity at heart and stick to the basics. Remember, *"physical training is of some value"* so let us apply it with purity in our lives. A little can go a long way, allowing you to focus on the more valuable areas in your life without getting carried away (more on these in chapter 6).

"Ok," you may ask, "but what does this look like?" Here are a few examples I share with my personal clients:

1. Organize a walking routine

> Whether indoor, on a hiking trail, or in your neighborhood set a day and time in your weekly schedule. Start small with 5-minutes and watch a new habit evolve. It's all about building a consistent routine as a building block to your wellness. You can get creative: short on time? Use walking as a devotional time between you and God. He deserves it and longs to fellowship with you.

2. Join a team sport

> Soccer leagues, softball, tennis, basketball, volleyball— the options are endless. Building a community around your activity helps with

consistency and support in the long run! *You were built for community.*

3. Add an active hobby

Pick up a new hobby like bike riding, hiking, swimming, golf (no cart), or kickboxing as a great way to stay moving. The more you are outdoors and breathing in fresh air the better. This can help melt away stress and allow you to "be in the moment."

4. Movement Therapy™

This is a term I have coined and implemented into my sessions with clients. It can be a form of intentional "yoga," rehab, corrective exercise, or active stretching which can lead you to preventing pain and injury while improving mobility. Movement Therapy includes specific, customized movements to help slow things down and move your body in new ways, releasing tension and stress, while activating key muscles. It could be as simple as building a small active-stretching routine you can apply daily to your life. Here are a few movements that promote healthy mobility:

Straight Leg Raises: this is great for releasing the hamstrings, activating the core, and protecting the lower back. Start on your back with both knees bent. You will then straighten one leg out, lift it up to your maximum range of motion, then lower down to the floor. Repeat for a few reps, about 10, and then switch.

During this movement, focus on your breath and keep the working leg straight to activate your quad (thigh) and core, in turn allowing your hamstrings to relax. 10 reps of 2 sets each leg would be a great start.

Seated Trunk Rotation with Extension: this is great for your mid-back, shoulders, and neck. Start in a seated chair position and practice rotating to your left and right (maximum ranges of motion) with your arms crossed over your chest. Stay mindful of your breathing. Once you reach your full turn to one side, slowly stretch down (as if crunching), and then while staying turned, activate your back by extending upward back to sitting position. Repeat on both sides for a few reps. 5 reps of 2 sets each side would be a great start. *Retest at the end to see if you've improved your rotation!*

Seated Trunk Side Bend: this is one of my favorites and great for those with lower or mid-back pain/tightness. You will start in a seated chair or bed position. Cross your arms over your chest, then slowly breathe out while crunching to one side a few times. Then repeat to the other side. Just make sure to stay mindful and move slow. 5 reps of 2 sets each side will yield beneficial results.

5. Build a resistance training routine

Weighted exercise comes with many benefits such as improved bone density, mood, and muscle mass. As you age, bone density and muscle mass become more valuable for long life and vitality. Resistance training is the gold standard but choose what you enjoy.

Everyone is different, and you don't have to do what others do or sign up for a gym membership to get active. I personally enjoy body weight exercises, resistance bands, and free weights— such as kettlebells.

Here is an example of a circuit training routine I created for efficiency and preventing injury to use with my clients. It encompasses a full body approach, while staying mindful of posture and balancing exercises to promote mobility and well-being (not just another "killer" workout). If you don't know the exercise, use your friendly search engine (such as Google) to help.

I call it Corrective Circuit Training™

1. *Resistance Band Row - 12 reps*
2. *Dumbbell Goblet Squat - 12 reps*
3. *Plank Hold - 30 seconds*
4. *Jumping Jacks - 20 reps*

Perform 4 rounds, with minimal rest. Challenge yourself, get creative, and have fun in 20 minutes or less. If you try this workout, post about it on Instagram and tag me @360wellness for a feature!

I encourage you to explore something new from these 5 examples above and write down ways you can apply it to your life. Today!

Every day is a new day. You have so much to enjoy and be thankful for, including the freedom to move. This calls for gratitude. *From God alone, you are given another day to breathe, move, and enjoy life with others.* You must stay reminded of the humility in all of this. Thankfulness for another day goes a long way and taking a walk to remember your purpose sure beats stressing out about your image or the thoughts of others.

Remember, if you take care of the inside, the outside will reflect.

Today's culture is begging for you to give into self-consciousness and ego. Don't believe the lies. You must step away from these negative thoughts and receive God's love for yourself daily. He is what matters most. Not our six-pack, the amount of likes we get on social media, or even who we date or marry will ever outweigh this truth of His abundant love.

In turn, through honoring your body, caring for it to promote health and well-being, you can reverse and prevent many forms of sickness and disease. Not to mention, you can live a happier and more capable life. I'm convinced that in the world today, with all the luxury (compared to third-world countries) and limited activity in our jobs or school, you must constantly be proactive with your health, and for the right reasons.

You have an opportunity today to respond, not merely listen. In the U.S., a sedentary lifestyle will only become more common as technology increases. If you don't build healthy exercise habits now, you may pay the bigger price later. No longer can you rely on your job or daily to-do list to ensure your strength and longevity as our ancestors once did. Believers must be examples of strength and discipline in every area of our life. This is "mind over matter. And matter over mind." How you handle and challenge your physical self affects your mind and spirit, and vice versa.

2 Timothy 1:7 AMP, *"For God did not give us a spirit of timidity or cowardice or fear, but [He has given us a spirit] of power and of love and of sound judgment and*

> *personal discipline [abilities that result in a calm, well-balanced mind and self-control]."*

Lastly, the concept of mental toughness has been on my heart. Exercise can also be used as a tool to build mental strength and self-discipline. There is truth to this, and as the world indulges in "easy," it would be wise to challenge your comfort zone and resist the temptation of laziness, even "sloth."

There's a saying that goes, "If you're not growing, you're dying." As a Believer you need to challenge your body, mind, and spirit daily to ensure growth to be your best. *Discomfort is what builds greatness.* You don't grow by being comfortable, and you don't get a diamond without a little pressure. Whatever way you want to look at it, step back and consider how you can apply exercise to start challenging your comfort zone.

Christians should be some of the healthiest people on earth, setting an example of wellness for the world. Imagine if you walked out your life with active intention, challenging yourself daily in all areas, while staying strong (physically and mentally) to impact the lives of others. Can you imagine yourself now? Take a moment. What would that look like to you?

What if you lived to be a giver and a solid foundation to those in need, even into old age? Exercise may attribute to a small portion in this equation, but it's still a portion. Do not neglect your body. You are only given one.

Lastly, I don't know who this is for but it's hard and I understand. *Life gets thrown at you, yet don't let the excuse of denying the flesh empower yourself to neglect God's temple.* There is a difference between caring for the body God has given you and denying yourself. It may be a thin line, but you must acknowledge this: no longer can we continue allowing pain, injury, sickness, and the like to occur just because we were not good stewards of our own body. Sometimes it's not spiritual warfare, it's just you. We are all capable of becoming our worst enemy.

So, I challenge you now. *Utilize your time today, start your new season, and continue moving forward to grow into the full potential God has given you.* It could start with a simple practice such as "making the time" for that 5-minute workout, organizing your health as a priority, or going the extra mile to care for someone in need (even when you're busy).

In the next chapter, you will discover just how you can gain greater control over your lifestyle, continue to prevent health issues, and make conscious, mindful, self-controlled choices to be your best. And it starts with the power of *nutrition.*

Reflect

What would your life look like if you lived with active intention and challenged yourself daily in all areas to impact the lives of others? If you lived to be 120, what do you want to be known for? How will you begin to set an active, healthy foundation in your life today?

Chapter IV – Nutrition

1 Peter 5:8 AMP, *"Be sober [well balanced and self-disciplined], be alert and cautious at all times. That enemy of yours, the devil, prowls around like a roaring lion [fiercely hungry], seeking someone to devour."*

Nutrition is your foundation. From your physical, mental, to spiritual self, sound nutrition stands strong as a leader in health and transformation. Let me explain.

If you think about eating and satisfying the body (flesh), they can go hand in hand. It is our most basic and primitive action. *What you consume and why you consume matters.* Yet, it's often the one thing Believers, pastors, and missionaries "let go" or overlook. I've seen it time and time again, even experiencing it myself— especially on mission trips. We tend to be comfortable with "getting everything else right" while letting our diet suffer because we "deserve it" or we think, "what's the harm" (when there's grace)?

We are missing an opportunity here. Many of you know the power of fasting in your prayer life and the positive effect it has in your walk as a Believer. After fasting from food, however, you tend to go back to living as you did before. It's normal. Yet, it's this inconsistent way of life I challenge you on. What if you practiced setting aside your desires and denied certain eating and drinking habits that hinder your spiritual potential consistently? In doing this, I believe the holistic benefits of "fasting" could be more continual and long-term.

Or maybe you have never practiced fasting before. Wherever you are at, I would like to introduce a new thought. *When you slow down and set your focus on nutrition as a priority, your life will change.* Whether you are a student, business executive, working mom, pastor, missionary, nutrition expert, or a combination, healthy habits go a long way in promoting not only the vitality of the body and mental health, but also spiritual clarity.

I think of healthy eating primarily as *self-control and self-care.* Applying these as spiritual practices to your diet feeds into your daily lifestyle, as well as your relationship with God (no pun intended). It's not that fasting, or self-denial brings us any closer to God, but that we clear the distractions or "static" of the flesh, for the flesh and the Spirit are in opposition.

> Galatians 5:17 AMP, *"For the sinful nature has its desire which is opposed to the Spirit, and the [desire of the] Spirit opposes the sinful nature; for these [two, the sinful nature and the Spirit] are in direct opposition to each other [continually in conflict], so that you [as believers] do not [always] do whatever [good things] you want to do."*

When you are constantly feeding (literally) every want and need of the flesh, it can seep into other areas of your life. Sin always starts subtle. We must stay "alert and cautious" (1 Peter 5:8) to live a life of purity and consistency for the Kingdom. Christ was sent to restore your spirit, why squander it?

> Romans 8:3-4 AMP, *"For what the Law could not do [that is, overcome sin and remove its penalty, its power] being weakened by the flesh [man's nature without the Holy Spirit], God did: He sent His own Son in the likeness of sinful man as an offering for sin. And He*

condemned sin in the flesh [subdued it and overcame it in the person of His own Son], so that the [righteous and just] requirement of the Law might be fulfilled in us who do not live our lives in the ways of the flesh [guided by worldliness and our sinful nature], but [live our lives] in the ways of the Spirit [guided by His power]."

Please hang with me here. Practically, for example, sugar or similar "ultra-flavor foods" (e.g., salty/savory) are known to be "addictive," almost "irresistible" by design – or at the very least have an influence on your behavior through chemicals in your brain. A small amount of influence goes farther than you think.

Regardless of choice, this influence (or effect) changes the way you think, and therefore act. Back in 2016, during a time I had in prayer with God, I came to a revelation while I myself was struggling with eating habits along with on and off depression:

"If everything is a choice, including loving God, then eating foods that hinder our choices probably isn't a good idea."

Read that one more time. Love is a choice. The scriptures have always called you to *action*. There is grace, but God wants you to step out in faith. Even when you try your best (which will never be enough) the Lord's grace catches you, filling in what you never could because He loves you. This is relationship. This is unconditional love.

Matthew 22:37 AMP, *"And Jesus replied to him, 'You shall love the Lord your God with all your heart, and with all your soul, and with all your mind.'"*

1 Corinthians 8:3 AMP, *"But if anyone loves God [with awe-filled reverence, obedience and gratitude], he is known by Him [as His very own and is greatly loved]."*

1 John 4:21 AMP, *"And this commandment we have from Him, that the one who loves God should also [unselfishly] love his brother and seek the best for him."*

1 John 5:2 AMP, *"By this we know [without any doubt] that we love the children of God: [expressing that love] when we love God and obey His commandments."*

All these scriptures state love as a verb.

Now, back to my story. Again, in 2016 when I was working as a personal trainer and sports massage therapist with a passion for nutrition, I became surprised when I saw how food impacted my everyday behavior. Although I was just beginning my journey into business and my relationship with God was deepening, I had continued revelations that branched off the "sugar" topic.

I was going through up and down depression, along with seasons of poor food and lifestyle choices. I just wasn't thinking straight or consistently. I knew this wasn't me, and it wasn't from God. As we know from scripture, we can battle against spiritual warfare (the devil/demons), our flesh (sinful nature), and the world (sinful culture). This was one of those times I could feel it was a combination. My flesh was getting in the way, and I felt the enemy was using it against me while I was genuinely seeking God.

There are many tactics the enemy can use against you that rarely seem "demonic," but you must not forget the devil is subtle and crafty. If he can't beat you, he sure can try to confuse and attack your mind. This is one reason why I am so passionate about nutrition. I see a lot of the mental health battles people go through today actually being caused from a poor diet, yet we call it "mental health issues."

From that point forward, I felt led to go on a fast. Not just any fast, but one that removed common indulging and satisfying food and drink. From my scientific background, you could say all things that released high levels of dopamine.

What is *dopamine*?

A quote from <u>Into Action Recovery Center</u> describes dopamine as "one of the 'feel good' chemicals in our brain. Interacting with the pleasure and reward center of our brain, dopamine — along with other chemicals like serotonin, oxytocin, and endorphins — plays a vital role in how happy we feel. In addition to our mood, dopamine also affects movement, memory, and focus. Healthy levels of dopamine drive us to seek and repeat pleasurable activities, while low levels can have an adverse physical and psychological impact."

They go on to say, "imbalances in these chemicals impact our behavior and quality of life and can create a vast amount of health issues," including a list below:

- Anxiety
- Addiction
- Behavioral disturbances
- Cognitive disorders
- Diseases (Such as Parkinson's)
- Fatigue
- Hormonal imbalances
- Mood disorders
- Obesity
- Pain

This is where science and faith meet. Isn't God good? Some things in the Bible are meant for our own good, whether we realize it or not. After doing my research, I began making a list of everything that can influence you in this way to an unhealthy degree.

I came up with these 7:

- Added Sugar
- Smoking/Drugs
- Social Media
- Highly Processed Foods
- Caffeine
- Sexual Relations
- Alcohol

These 7 stood out to me as the most common and influential factors we deal with today. A week after I wrote about these things in my notebook, something happened. While I was in prayer, I heard the Lord speak to my heart (I always describe receiving a Word as an overriding thought):

"I want you to fast of these things, until Sunday the 19th."
(Key word Sunday)

I reacted thinking, "Pshh, last week was the 19th. This wasn't from God."

Yeah, last week was the 19th. It seemed God wanted me to fast from these things for three full weeks. I checked the calendar, and sure enough the 19th of the following month fell on a Sunday (it happened to be exactly 21 days) to solidify my belief. Crazy? Well, God knows your heart and can speak to it. Sometimes you just have to be still and listen.

I have concluded that whenever there is an important shift or transition in my life or around it, God encourages me to fast. It may be for unseen reasons, but I also know from experience, it heightens my sensitivity to Him, limiting the flesh that can get in the way. His ways are always higher than mine (Isaiah 55:8-9).

The bottom line: fasting cleanses your body, mind, and spirit by limiting the flesh and empowering the Spirit. I always sense and hear God more clearly during a fast and have heard the same from others.

This basically left me with water, whole foods, and the Bible (I don't recommend eating your Bible). Believe me, the first few days were not easy (and I mean NOT EASY), but after that, something opened up. It's amazing the control these factors can have over your life, yet rarely do you realize it.

During my fast, I experienced an increase in clarity, focus, energy, motivation, and self-control. I had never felt better! *God was showing me the powerful effects a healthy diet and lifestyle could have on my life and in turn those around me.* He wants us to shine bright. And so, I want to share this secret with you.

I call it the **21 Day: Dopamine Fast**. As mentioned above, you will cut out these pleasurable foods, drinks, and habits for 21 days (get ready for the fun!). Trust me, you will not regret it. This can be used as an annual reset for the body, mind, and spirit or as a consistent lifestyle change you create to thrive in the Spirit and in life.

The official list is as follows:

1. Added Sugar (all kinds e.g., honey, white, brown, organic "super-sugar")
2. Smoking/Drugs (cigarettes, marijuana etc.)
3. Social Media (Facebook, Instagram, Twitter etc.)

4. Processed Foods (non-sprouted bread, cheese, chips etc.)
5. Caffeine (coffee, green tea etc.)
6. Sexual Relations
7. Alcohol

If you feel that cutting these out all at once is too much to handle, I understand. I recommend you make a swift change for best results but choosing one area to focus on each week and building from there works as well. In that case, I would encourage you to start with the easiest choice and work toward your most challenging. This will allow you to build momentum and healthy habits that hopefully will last once the 21 days are over.

You may not deal with all 7 of these areas so if one doesn't apply to you, great! No matter the number of factors you choose, work toward 21 days and let yourself reset. *Your body, mind, and spirit will thank you and I believe God will reward your faithfulness during this season.* Abide in Him during this time, and you will not fail.

Yes, it will not be easy, and the flesh is weak, but if this fast feels like the right choice for you, I encourage you to *pray*. Ask God for the strength and grace needed during this time. You must remember in our weakness, He is strong, and it's not by your own strength but by His Spirit (Zechariah 4:6).

The main purpose of this fast is to help you reset and take back control of your thoughts, feelings, actions, and emotions that may have been affected by a poor diet, social media, and other behaviors. This is different from your average fast in which you abstain from food for a few days. This practice is meant to integrate into your daily life, boosting your self-control and giving to God as an act of worship by denying the flesh (Romans

12:1). *This is where the body, mind, and spirit intersect, as one truly affects the other.*

From there, you can more easily transition into a consistently healthy lifestyle with fewer cravings, choosing to manage your diet the way you want to and maximizing your health for the long run. You will also experience greater energy, focus, and have a more positive outlook on life! If you are looking for coaching or more direction on this practice, please visit http://the360wellness.com

There's one last factor I would like to discuss specifically. *Caffeine.* Coffee is one of the leading drinks in the world that keeps us going. "It keeps the world turning" you might say. Throughout my personal experience of the 21-day fast, I was surprised by how much I relied on coffee for energy. In the morning, in the afternoon, it was part of my daily routine. When I cut it out, I began withdrawals as an addict would experience when removing their drug from their life. Headaches, depression, lack of motivation, mental fog, irritation, and the like all followed as I cut caffeine out of my life. Is this the way it's supposed to be?

I challenge your thinking today. Does caffeine have some benefits? Of course. I see it as a tool, but as I walked into day 4, day 5, day 6, of the fast I realized that *food*, yes food, was my supplier of energy. I had to eat 4-5 medium sized meals to keep up with my activity and work demands without caffeine. And do you know what? I felt GREAT. No longer was I slave to a substance I idolized for so long. The Lord gave you the sweet blessing of food and He has not called you to be slave to any man or thing, yet I see so many of us captured (or even addicted) by this simple ingredient.

Romans 6:15-18 AMP, *"What then [are we to conclude]? Shall we sin because we are not under Law, but under [God's] grace? Certainly not! Do you not know that when you continually offer yourselves to someone to do his will, you are the slaves of the one whom you obey, either [slaves] of sin, which leads to death, or of obedience, which leads to righteousness (right standing with God)? But thank God that though you were slaves of sin, you became obedient with all your heart to the standard of teaching in which you were instructed and to which you were committed. And having been set free from sin, you have become the slaves of righteousness [of conformity to God's will and purpose]."*

So, I call you out of that place. *As a child of God, I call you to overcome even the little things holding you back from fully walking in complete sonship to the Father.* He is our Rock. He is our Source. Let us never forget this and be distracted by the lusts of this world that seem so innocent. Give the devil no foothold for you are called to walk with power, discipline, and authority by grace, constantly attaining the mind of Christ and having God first and foremost in your life.

This revelation sums up my thoughts on the power of food and the effects it can have on us. Am I perfect with all of this? Believe me, I am not. If someone brings in some doughnuts… sign me up! However, when I indulge and give way to the flesh and its desires, I know ultimately the effect it can have on me. I have seen the other side. When I slow down, reframe, and look ahead toward my long-term goals, I can break the temptations that only lead to short-term satisfaction. Over time it gets easier and easier. When you stay consistent, a kind of resilience builds up. Just like when you exercise, your muscles initially break down, yet you come back stronger.

Now, let me be clear, I'm not saying processed foods, sugar, alcohol, and the like are "bad." I believe in balance, moderation, and a healthy relationship with these things. However, I also think it's important to be aware of your intentions, checking your heart, and knowing the negative side effects of these choices, which are so readily available. There is no such thing as a "bad" food and food does not defile you. It's the why behind it.

> Mark 7:15 AMP, *"there is nothing outside a man [such as food] which by going into him can defile him [morally or spiritually]; but the things which come out of [the heart of] a man are what defile and dishonor him."*

I know there is talk about distrust of the food and drink industry, along with the social media, and how it can seem to be against us, causing sickness, obesity, depression, and anxiety. We like to play the blame game, and this may be true in some instances. Maybe certain leaders in the industries are all about making money and marketing products regardless of the impact on our physical and mental health.

But from personal experience, and what I believe God has shown me, I challenge you to look at things a little differently. YOU. Yes, you are ultimately in control. I encourage you to hold every thought (and action) captive in your life. If you have to delete social media, then delete it. If you need to keep junk food out of your kitchen, then do it. There's a saying from Precision Nutrition co-founder and CEO, John Berardi, which goes something like this, "If a food is in your house or possession, either you, someone you love, or someone you marginally tolerate will eventually eat it." This is just human psychology.

And what does Jesus say about temptation?

> Matthew 5:30 AMP, *"If your right hand makes you stumble and leads you to sin, cut it off and throw it away [that is, remove yourself from the source of temptation]; for it is better for you to lose one of the parts of your body than for your whole body to go into hell."*

Again, the flesh is weak, but the spirit is willing. God is stronger. This may be a fluid process with highs and lows, but I believe in you. Continually keep moving forward and let the grace of God daily into your life to attain the mind of Christ in all you do. Amen.

> Matthew 26:41 AMP, *"Keep actively watching and praying that you may not come into temptation; the spirit is willing, but the body is weak."*

> *1* Corinthians 2:16 AMP, *"For WHO HAS KNOWN THE MIND and PURPOSES OF THE LORD, SO AS TO INSTRUCT HIM? But we have the mind of Christ [to be guided by His thoughts and purposes]."*

For example, can you see Jesus going to a party and indulging in all the chips? Probably not. Can you see Jesus struggling with His Starbucks or Instagram addiction? It's a bit funny to even think about... I don't think so. *He was fully centered in who He was and although tempted as you are, did not give into the lust of the world.* The enemy is subtle, and every sinful habit starts small. As Damon Thompson, worldwide revivalist, calls it, "one lamb at a time" based on shepherding in the scriptures.

> *Don't give in to the little things, and you can prevent the greater.*

You may say, "But my work is so stressful and busy. I don't have time to eat healthy!" That is fair. I understand there is a need for work and responsibilities take a priority. But is that really worth your mental health or the potential of a full relationship with God? Jesus says it Himself in Mark 8:36 (AMP).

> *"For what does it benefit a man to gain the whole world [with all its pleasures], and forfeit his soul?"*

This is just food for thought (geez really with the puns). I do not mean to overload you, but there is truly power in sound nutrition. All you have to do is start making small adjustments to your health, and I promise you, it doesn't take as much energy or time as you think. In fact, it will give you more.

I heard a saying the other day that goes something like this,

> "Most people spend their health seeking wealth, to then only end up spending their wealth seeking health."

Health truly is wealth. When you believe and walk out on these truths, you empower yourself through Christ to rise above the world's mentality. No longer are you walking in the way of the world, but you have taken a narrow path. It may be lonely and against the grain, but it produces life for the present and the life to come (1 Timothy 4:8).

You may say, "But it's everywhere! I feel like it is inevitable." Or "I grew up with it. It's a part of my culture."

Welcome to Jesus culture. Take every thought captive, beloved. If you are serious about change then setting goals, setting plans, setting small daily actions, and setting up your environment for success are your keys to move against the grain of influence. Below are some prompts to help you write it out, putting pen to paper, and thoughts to action!

1. Mindset

What can you set your mind on today? *Through Christ you have the fruit of the Spirit: love, joy, peace, patience, kindness, goodness, faithfulness, gentleness, and self-control* (Galatians 5:22-23). In the Spirit, you attain these.

So, on all occasions remind yourself of these truths; write them out, pray them over yourself, even when you don't "feel like it." Emotions come and go, but God is truth. This is about conquering the flesh. Your identity is in Him, always.

2. Goals

What does healthy eating or a healthy lifestyle look like to you? What do you want to improve but haven't in your life? For example, this could be anywhere from losing 20 pounds, to improving your mental health.

3. Plan

How are you going to do it? What skills or practices do you need to accomplish your goal/s? For example, you want to cook at home. A *practice* would be weekly grocery shopping.

4. Small actions

Now break those practices down. What are a few things you can easily do *daily* to set yourself up for success? For example, setting a timer to remind yourself to drink water or marking your to-dos in your calendar the night before.

5. Environment

Set up your kitchen, workplace, and community to empower the type of goals you want to achieve. How can you stay consistent if you have a lot of junk food around and your gym bag or running shoes are tucked away somewhere? The better your environment is set up for your health, the greater chance you have of accomplishing short-term and long-term goals. This is sometimes overlooked. Clear out the *roadblocks*. Think ahead!

Does your kitchen, workflow, and community/friends support your goals? Check. You may be surprised. Write down potential roadblocks that may get in the way, along with adjustments you could make in your environment to support this.

Once these are in place, start by adding *more* fresh, whole, less-processed foods to your diet. Think "whole" foods defined as a single ingredient. This includes all fruits, vegetables, fish, nuts, beans, rice, and the like. By integrating these consistently into your diet over highly processed foods (junk food), you've taken a huge step in prevention from sickness, disease, inflammation, and poor mental health. Make it fun. Mix it up. Explore new foods.

To start you off, here are 5 easy ways to apply healthy nutrition to your routine:

1. Plan, prioritize, and prepare

Make it easy on yourself. Try meal prepping in advance for three days at a time (or a certain meal daily like breakfast), picking up premade meals at your local grocery store, or even try a meal delivery system. There are lots of options out there these days!

Choose what works best for you and your budget. Remember, you can't take healthy action if you're not set up to do it.

2. Quality over quantity

The better quality of food or drink you can choose the better. This has been shown to improve digestion, provide more nutrients, and improve satisfaction. Also, you can usually eat more while taking in less calories if the food is whole and high quality as opposed to refined and processed.

Less is more in this situation.

3. Drink water, silly

What can I say, water makes up around 55-60% of who you are! But did you know that a large percent of the U.S. population is chronically dehydrated? I recommend starting with 12 cups a day for men, and 10 cups a day for women. See how it works for you (some may need more or less - depending on body type).

I know there are some people who don't like plain water. That's ok, let's think creatively. Add lemon. Drink low calorie tea or carbonated water. There's a positive impact to your health if you consistently hydrate.

Proper hydration eases strain on the heart, boosts physical and mental performance, cleanses kidneys, and even helps maintain hormone balance.

4. Eat a salad-a-day

I can't emphasize enough how healthy raw vegetables are for you. They supply you with important fiber and probiotics to support gut-health which are key to overall health and vitality. That is why I recommend a salad a day (at least). Get creative, find what you like, and plan to apply it this week.

I'm personally big on "hearty" salads, incorporating lean protein, such as fish or boiled eggs and healthy carbs, such as quinoa or black beans.

5. Practice mindful eating

Slow down. Honestly, this is my most difficult practice. In the past, I would tend to eat fast (I always blamed it on not wanting my food to get cold). Research, however, has found multiple benefits in slowing down, enjoying, and being mindful of every bite. These include better digestion, consuming less, and higher satisfaction after eating.

Are you up for trying it during your next meal? You may be surprised with the results!

In terms of health and nutrition, we all tend to know during this day and age what is healthy or unhealthy. "Eat more vegetables, less cotton candy. Got it." In life, you usually know WHAT to do, you just don't DO it. The 5 steps above will help you take action and stay consistent along the way (the key to long-term health and prevention).

Lastly, is the idea *of nutrition and self-care*. I see nutrition as a reflection of loving and fueling your body, or in other words, tending to your temple (God's temple). Many of us have a poor relationship with food, but maybe we just need to adjust our perspective. Food is life. It nourishes, supplies, and supports your body to live life to the fullest. You have a choice.

You can love your body in a way that lets you find long-term satisfaction in living your best life for God, or you can overindulge and let the blessing of having food on your table hinder your full potential (in body, mind, and spirit).

Many of you are blessed to have enough food on the table, yet, around the world people live day-to-day hoping to just get enough (while others over consume). I think we are called to withhold from this indulging way of life. Imagine if you began to eat just what you needed to nourish your body and gave the rest to those in need. There would be *change*. There would be *impact*.

A saying I always saw in my kitchen growing up as a kid stuck with me. It goes something like this,

"Live simply, so others can simply live."

As I have said before, this way of life will not be easy, and I am working on this area myself. However, mature growth as Believers is uncomfortable and in opposition to the ways of the world. It is up to you to make the conscious choice. Not because you have to, there is grace, but because this will allow your greatness to begin to unfold for God's glory, so you can maximize your time on earth and love others fully.

After all, you are called to be the light, exposing darkness with your actions and character.

Ephesians 5:14-18 AMP, *"For this reason He says, 'Awake, sleeper, And arise from the dead, And Christ will shine [as dawn] upon you and give you light.' Therefore see that you walk carefully [living life with honor, purpose, and courage; shunning those who tolerate and enable evil], not as the unwise, but as wise [sensible, intelligent, discerning people], making the very most of your time [on earth, recognizing and taking advantage of each opportunity and using it with wisdom and diligence], because the days are [filled with] evil. Therefore do not be foolish and thoughtless, but understand and firmly grasp what the will of the Lord is. Do not get drunk with wine, for that is wickedness (corruption, stupidity), but be filled with the [Holy] Spirit and constantly guided by Him."*

You must live a life of awareness and diligence, discerning the negative influence all around you, and choosing to be proactive before it is too late because the days are evil.

Often, we are pushed and pulled through life, "asleep," not even noticing the poor habits we are building or hindering choices that we are making. Therefore, we must take notice. This calls for *mindfulness*.

Reflect

What does healthy eating or a healthy lifestyle look like to you? What do you want to improve in your life and how are you going to do it? What are a few things you can easily do daily to set yourself up for success?

Chapter V – Mindfulness

Isaiah 26: 3 AMP, *"You will keep in perfect and constant peace the one whose mind is steadfast [that is, committed and focused on You—in both inclination and character], because he trusts and takes refuge in You [with hope and confident expectation]."*

What do you think of when you hear *"mindfulness?"*

Over the years, I have worked to improve mine. I see the importance of it in everything I do, whether I'm hanging out with family, working, or becoming still to pray. It is something I have begun to integrate into every area of my life.

According to Oxford Dictionary, mindfulness is "a mental state achieved by focusing one's awareness on the present moment." This practice can be integrated into everything you do. I love Brené Brown's description of mindfulness in her best-selling book, *Dare to Lead.*

She calls it *"Paying attention."* It's simple, yet powerful.

When I started working as a personal trainer in 2014, I noticed something my clients had in common. They were not in-tune with or aware of their own body. This pattern continued to surface as I began working with therapy clients who were in pain or had experienced injury, and even continued to show up in my coaching and nutrition clients. Most of the time, they were unaware of their posture, poor movement, and/or exactly what they were putting into their bodies through diet (and how it was affecting them). I think it's safe to say, as humans, we tend to struggle with focus and that's what I want to bring to your attention throughout this chapter.

In addition to adding a consistent focus on recovery, exercise, and nutrition to your life, mindfulness is vital. Let's be honest, it's challenging to be in the present moment on any given day. Our world makes it easy to stay distracted. We are constantly bombarded with texts, emails, notifications, commercials, ads, and to-dos. Our focus is constantly being challenged, even worn-down.

This needs to change. You need to reclaim your daily focus by conserving energy, concentrating your efforts toward growth, and staying in the moment. For example, notice your posture right now! Are you slouching? (I was)

To start, I've provided my top 5 tips to encourage daily mindfulness:

1. Set a daily reminder

Set a time when you know you are busy to stop, breath, practice gratitude, or whatever works for you to reset and be in the moment. The 21st century calls for your attention, constantly pulling you away from peace, thankfulness, and contentment. *Use this practice to stop and find peace, His peace.*

2. Focus on one thing at a time

Most of us juggle tasks throughout the day and feel good about it. Yet, concentrating your focus on one thing at a time can help you not only perform the task better, but also enjoy the moment (and with less stress). That could be reading this book, playing with your children, working on a school assignment, or exercising at the gym.

Whatever it is, use your precious time, energy, and focus wisely. Our time on earth is short, so let's make the most of it.

Focus.

3. Perform a mind-body scan

This technique helps you center yourself to be in the moment. I like to add this in the morning during my prayer time with God. You can start at the top of your head, working down to your feet, noticing and relaxing each part of your body as you breath in-and-out. It may feel funny at first, but this truly works and can help you to relax as it releases tension from your body.

4. Practice active listening

This means to engage in your conversations, not thinking about what you are going to say next but practicing truly hearing whoever is speaking. Notice the little things, staying in the moment, remembering they are children of God. *Lost or found.*

This is the beginning of empathy and compassion.

5. *Meditating on the Word*

Set a time to read, meditate, and pray in private, just you and God. It could be first thing in the morning, at night before bed, or even during your lunch break in your car. When you carve out and make the time it becomes special. It shows intention and diligence, while being a form of worship in and of itself. Practice during your quiet time, shutting off all outside distractions (phone, email, and the like).

A favorite mindfulness centered passage to read:

Philippians 4:4-9, AMP, "*Rejoice in the Lord always [delight, take pleasure in Him]; again I will say, rejoice! Let your gentle spirit [your graciousness, unselfishness, mercy, tolerance, and patience] be known to all people. The Lord is near. Do not be anxious or worried about anything, but in everything [every circumstance and situation] by prayer and petition with thanksgiving, continue to make your [specific] requests known to God. 7 And the peace of God [that peace which reassures the heart, that peace] which transcends all understanding, [that peace which] stands guard over your hearts and your minds in Christ Jesus [is yours].*

Finally, believers, whatever is true, whatever is honorable and worthy of respect, whatever is right and confirmed by God's word, whatever is pure and wholesome, whatever is lovely and brings peace, whatever is admirable and of good repute; if there is any excellence, if there is anything worthy of praise, think continually on these things [center your mind on them, and implant them in your heart]. The things which you have learned and received and heard and seen in me, practice these things [in daily life], and the God [who is the source] of peace and well-being will be with you."

Just 5 minutes a day goes a long way, and something is always better than nothing. Meditate on His word and you will find life.

Now, to extend my thoughts on mindfulness, scripture tells us you are called to take every thought captive and to set your mind on the things above. Do not forget, your battle is often in the mind, not against each other.

2 Corinthians 10:5 AMP, *"We are destroying sophisticated arguments and every exalted and proud thing that sets itself up against the [true] knowledge of God, and we are taking every thought and purpose captive to the obedience of Christ..."*

Colossians 3:2 AMP, *"Set your mind and keep focused habitually on the things above [the heavenly things], not on things that are on the earth [which have only temporal value]."*

Ephesians 6:12 AMP, *"For our struggle is not against flesh and blood [contending only with physical opponents], but against the rulers, against the powers, against the world forces of this [present] darkness, against the spiritual forces of wickedness in the heavenly (supernatural) places."*

There is power in the mind, and what you focus on you empower. Because of this, you need to awaken from the "sleep" of stress, unproductive habits, and letting your environment control you. You are you. Perfectly and wonderfully made through Christ to be the *"head and not the tail."* I know you may not feel like this all the time, but it's not about how you feel. Feelings fade.

You were created to do great things, not for yourself, but for others. Imagine the great freedom and peace in this if you just believed it, even for a moment. Now, take a step back and remember your identity.

> Deuteronomy 28:13 AMP, *"The LORD will make you the head (leader) and not the tail (follower); and you will be above only, and you will not be beneath, if you listen and pay attention to the commandments of the LORD your God, which I am commanding you today, to observe them carefully."*

> Galatians 4:31 AMP, *"So then, believers, we [who are born again—reborn from above—spiritually transformed, renewed, and set apart for His purpose] are not children of a slave woman [the natural], but of the free woman [the supernatural]."*

> Galatians 5:1 AMP, *"It was for this freedom that Christ set us free [completely liberating us]; therefore keep standing firm and do not be subject again to a yoke of slavery [which you once removed]."*

What if you began to take the time to be consistently intentional with your thoughts and your life? What would change if you paid attention to every area of life, staying in the moment? How would your life shift if you constantly meditated on the Word of God and the truth of your identity in Christ?

I believe your life would change. Imagine yourself mentally stronger, more focused, happier, and driven. This is exactly what the enemy doesn't want. *He doesn't want you walking in the constant mindfulness of who you are to God, and the power of freedom that Christ has given you.* Remember your struggle is not against flesh and blood (Ephesians 6:12), there are things, both seen and unseen, pulling you away from the mind of Christ. You must begin to learn how to recognize and identify these areas in your life.

I remember hearing a sermon by Dan Mohler on Adam and Eve regarding *identity*. Whether you believe this to be a parable or a historical event, it holds meaning and truth. Here is the passage from Genesis 3:1-4 AMP:

Now the serpent was more crafty (subtle, skilled in deceit) than any living creature of the field which the LORD God had made. And the serpent (Satan) said to the woman, "Can it really be that God has said, 'You shall not eat from any tree of the garden'?" And the woman said to the serpent, "We may eat fruit from the trees of the garden, except the fruit from the tree which is in the middle of the garden. God said, 'You shall not eat from it nor touch it, otherwise you will die.'" But the serpent said to the woman, "You certainly will not die! For God knows that on the day you eat from it your eyes will be opened [that is, you will have greater awareness], and you will be like God, knowing [the difference between] good and evil."

Mohler interpreted this passage as the snake (devil) tempting Eve, saying she would have great knowledge and awareness if she ate from the forbidden tree: that she would be like God. Adam and Eve, however, were already made in the image of God, fully whole and alive, having dominion on this earth (Genesis 1:26-28). Mohler concluded that since the beginning the devil has been trying to shift your mind, causing you to forget who you are (causing your spirit to die in separation from God) and in turn, forgetting what you are here on this earth to do. Take dominion with love while walking with God.

The world can have you stressed and focused on the wrong things, but they don't bring life because they are not Truth. They only feed the flesh and are often derived from fear (faith has no fear). You must re-center and refocus your mind to your true identity and the good things of God by being diligent with your thoughts, remembering who you are as a follower of Christ.

Daily.

Having said this, I want to introduce a few practical ways you can apply mindfulness to your life, focusing on the 5 foundational concepts discussed in this book. These are more than just concepts. They're *values*. You can't have one without the others for complete holistic health.

Here are the 5:

1. Recovery

How are you feeling today? Are you tired? Happy? Dealing with pain? Stressed? Take a moment and write down how you are doing.

2. Exercise

When walking outdoors, exercising at the gym, or enjoying your favorite active hobby, are you in the moment? Are you noticing your stride, your posture, your energy levels? Make a note or set a reminder for your next exercise session and practice mindful movement, taking a break from your "to-do list," even for a moment.

3. Nutrition

Are you eating mindfully and with care? How does your food taste? What is the texture? Are you hungry? Would you feed what you're eating to your child? These are just some questions you can ask yourself at each meal. Take a minute and reflect.

Tip: mindful eating not only provides the health benefits discussed in chapter 4, but also allows you to enjoy your meals more, being in the moment with friends or family.

4. Mindfulness

It may be ironic to be mindful about mindfulness, but oh, it's a thing. Are you taking the time to write out your thoughts or journal? To take a deep breath? To stay in the moment and not jump ahead in your tasks? Do you practice taking every thought and action captive?

Write down one way you can stay more mindful or one thing you are grateful for at this time.

5. Faith

Do you not know who you are? As a believer in Jesus Christ, you are a child of God. Forgiven. Grafted into the vine. Adopted into the family. No longer are you forgotten or forsaken. No longer are you alone. No longer are you purposeless.

You now have trustworthy hope in the One whom we call Father. No matter your past, present, or future, you have a righteous all-powerful Father who loves you. Stay mindful of this. The faith and the hope we so carry in our spirit.

Proverbs 18:24b AMP, *"But there is a [true, loving] friend who [is reliable and] sticks closer than a brother."*

Next, we will look closer at the potential of your relationship with God and how faith integrates into wellness. This is the missing piece for those who are seeking wholeness.

Reflect

How would your life look if you were consistently intentional with your thoughts and your life? What would change if you paid attention to every area of life, staying in the moment? How might your life shift if you constantly meditated on the word of God and the truth of your identity in Christ?

Chapter VI – Faith

Luke 12:29-33 AMP, *"So as for you, do not seek what you will eat and what you will drink; nor have an anxious and unsettled mind. For all the [pagan] nations of the world greedily seek these things; and your [heavenly] Father [already] knows that you need them. But [strive for and actively] seek His kingdom, and these things will be given to you as well.*

Do not be afraid and anxious, little flock, for it is your Father's good pleasure to give you the kingdom. Sell your possessions (show compassion) and give [donations] to the poor. Provide money belts for yourselves that do not wear out, an unfailing and inexhaustible treasure in the heavens, where no thief comes near and no moth destroys. For where your treasure is, there your heart will be also."

Faith is untouchable. No one can steal it, and it cannot rust. It is a gift you don't deserve, but a tangible one you carry in your spirit through the Holy Spirit.

How does this apply to wellness? Well, in every way. As an industry, the fitness, health, and wellness fields have evolved from a single focus of the body (physical) to integrating focus of the mind (mental), but rarely have they touched on the spirit (spiritual). Certainly not a faith centered in Jesus Christ.

I want to assure you that times are changing. *God wants to pour out His Spirit into every professional field of this world,*

83

including healthcare. I believe without a doubt that you can't have complete health, wellness, and wholeness without *Faith.* It's what holds us together.

> Hebrews 11:1-2 NASB, *"Now faith is the assurance of things hoped for, the conviction of things not seen. For by it the men of old gained approval."*

> Colossians 1:16-17 AMP, *"For by Him all things were created in heaven and on earth, [things] visible and invisible, whether thrones or dominions or rulers or authorities; all things were created and exist through Him [that is, by His activity] and for Him. And He Himself existed and is before all things, and in Him all things hold together. [His is the controlling, cohesive force of the universe.]"*

When the situation isn't for you, but you have this feeling to keep trying. To believe in healing over your life although things look dim. To have peace in times of trial, focusing not on what you see but on the Word of God. To believe that if you continue to persist, you can overcome that addiction/sin. To believe that if God sent Christ... He loves you. *This is faith.*

There is power and healing in this unseen mentality. By incorporating the shield of faith into every aspect of your life you can walk boldly as a Believer, being the example that the world needs. You can be the head and not the tail because God wants a generation He can partner with for His glory. Life will not always bring what's expected, and things may not always look the way you want them to, but you are called to walk by faith, not by sight (2 Corinthians 5:7)

What if you added prayer to your daily situations, your injury or sickness, to those around you in need, or even into your business? Not only when you felt like it, but in faith according to

His word. *God wants to saturate every area of your life, yet naturally many of you tend to separate your faith from your daily life*. Your work. Your health. Your family.

Since the beginning, you were called to walk in the garden with Him daily, in all you do.

> Genesis 2:15 AMP, *"Then the LORD God took the man and put him into the garden of Eden to cultivate it and keep it."*

> Colossians 3:15-17 AMP, *"Let the peace of Christ [the inner calm of one who walks daily with Him] be the controlling factor in your hearts [deciding and settling questions that arise]. To this peace indeed you were called as members in one body [of believers].*

> *And be thankful [to God always]. Let the [spoken] word of Christ have its home within you [dwelling in your heart and mind—permeating every aspect of your being] as you teach [spiritual things] and admonish and train one another with all wisdom, singing psalms and hymns and spiritual songs with thankfulness in your hearts to God. Whatever you do [no matter what it is] in word or deed, do everything in the name of the Lord Jesus [and in dependence on Him], giving thanks to God the Father through Him."*

> Ephesians 6:18 AMP, *"With all prayer and petition pray [with specific requests] at all times [on every occasion and in every season] in the Spirit, and with this in view, stay alert with all perseverance and petition [interceding in prayer] for all God's people."*

The Bible is clear that God is and should be part of EVERY aspect of your life, including your daily lifestyle. This is the key to continual wholeness. You must abide in Him daily; it's what you were first and foremost created for (Deuteronomy 6:5). *Relationship.*

> Psalm 70:4 AMP, *"May all those who seek You [as life's first priority] rejoice and be glad in You; May those who love Your salvation say continually, "Let God be magnified!"*

> James 5:13-15 AMP, *"Is anyone among you suffering? He must pray. Is anyone joyful? He is to sing praises [to God]. Is anyone among you sick? He must call for the elders (spiritual leaders) of the church and they are to pray over him, anointing him with oil in the name of the Lord; and the prayer of faith will restore the one who is sick, and the Lord will raise him up; and if he has committed sins, he will be forgiven."*

These actions come through nothing else but faith. Do you have to live this out? Of course not. You have free will. However, I am here to empower your best self, to help you maximize your God-given potential so you can give your best in all you do. In other words, living a life of power, love, and freedom no matter the circumstances. This is my goal for you.

Paul wrote, while in jail, Philippians 4:10-12 (AMP),

> *"I rejoiced greatly in the Lord, that now at last you have renewed your concern for me; indeed, you were concerned about me before, but you had no opportunity to show it. Not that I speak from [any personal] need, for I have learned to be content [and self-sufficient through Christ, satisfied to the point where I am not disturbed or uneasy] regardless of my circumstances. I know how to get along and live humbly [in difficult times], and I also know how to enjoy abundance and live in prosperity. In*

any and every circumstance I have learned the secret [of
facing life], whether well-fed or going hungry, whether
having an abundance or being in need."

Christ is what satisfies. You can hide from the Truth or give in and pursue it with faith and love. I know God has created you for something great. It's just up to you to trust Him. To lean in. I believe in you, and that's why I've written this book. It's time for you to step into your destiny and impact the world, fully empowered by God.

For Jesus says in Matthew 5:14-16 AMP,

"You are the light of [Christ to] the world. A city set
on a hill cannot be hidden; nor does anyone light a lamp
and put it under a basket, but on a lampstand, and it
gives light to all who are in the house. Let your light
shine before men in such a way that they may see your
good deeds and moral excellence, and [recognize and
honor and] glorify your Father who is in heaven."

I pray that truth and clarity be given to you right now, in the name of Jesus Christ.

This is a calling, not a statement. You are created and destined for much and God loves you, truly sending His one and only Son to bring you back home to the Father.

So, I call out the greatness inside of you. You must take action, cutting out the distractions you can control. Pain, sickness, depression, anxiety, and obesity are not your calling and they must go. They are a distraction to your life that the world and sin have created.

The following scriptures define what's on my heart:

John 3:16-17 NASB, *"For God so loved the world, that He gave His only begotten Son, that whoever believes in Him shall not perish, but have eternal life. For God did not send the Son into the world to judge the world, but that the world might be saved through Him."*

Romans 8:15 NASB, *"For you have not received a spirit of slavery leading to fear again, but you have received a spirit of adoption as sons by which we cry out, 'Abba! Father!'"*

Through faith in Jesus Christ, you know He has taken your sinful place, and God now calls you "child." Adopted into a son or daughter relationship if you believe. *You are home.* The passage in Luke of the lost son exemplifies this. You were lost but now you are found.

Luke 15:11-32 NASB, *And He (Jesus) said, "A man had two sons. The younger of them said to his father, 'Father, give me the share of the estate that falls to me.' So he divided his wealth between them. And not many days later, the younger son gathered everything together and went on a journey into a distant country, and there he squandered his estate with loose living. Now when he had spent everything, a severe famine occurred in that country, and he began to be impoverished.*

So he went and hired himself out to one of the citizens of that country, and he sent him into his fields to feed swine. And he would have gladly filled his stomach with the pods that the swine were eating, and no one was giving anything to him. But when he came to his senses, he said, 'How many of my father's hired men have more than enough bread, but I am dying here with hunger! I will get up and go to my father, and will say to him,

*"Father, I have sinned against heaven, and in your sight;
I am no longer worthy to be called your son; make me as
one of your hired men."'*

*So he got up and came to his father. But while he was
still a long way off, his father saw him and felt
compassion for him, and ran and embraced him and
kissed him. And the son said to him, 'Father, I have
sinned against heaven and in your sight; I am no longer
worthy to be called your son.' But the father said to his
slaves, 'Quickly bring out the best robe and put it on him,
and put a ring on his hand and sandals on his feet; and
bring the fattened calf, kill it, and let us eat and
celebrate; for this son of mine was dead and has come to
life again; he was lost and has been found.' And they
began to celebrate. "Now his older son was in the field,
and when he came and approached the house, he heard
music and dancing. And he summoned one of the servants
and began inquiring what these things could be.*

*And he said to him, 'Your brother has come, and your
father has killed the fattened calf because he has received
him back safe and sound.' But he became angry and was
not willing to go in; and his father came out and began
pleading with him. But he answered and said to his
father, 'Look! For so many years I have been serving you
and I have never neglected a command of yours; and yet
you have never given me a young goat, so that I might
celebrate with my friends; but when this son of yours
came, who has devoured your wealth with prostitutes,
you killed the fattened calf for him.' And he said to him,
'Son, you have always been with me, and all that is mine
is yours. But we had to celebrate and rejoice, for this
brother of yours was dead and has begun to live, and was
lost and has been found.'"*

I hear the Father saying, *"You were made for me."* You. Were. Made. For. Me.

You were made to be a child again, the way it used to be, trusting and abiding in God, able to rest in the truth and the love of the presence the Father brings. You were made to walk in the garden, being guided and taught by Him daily. Everyone can experience the gift of a relationship with God now through Jesus Christ!

> Galatians 4:4-5 AMP, *"But when [in God's plan] the proper time had fully come, God sent His Son, born of a woman, born under the [regulations of the] Law, so that He might redeem and liberate those who were under the Law, that we [who believe] might be adopted as sons [as God's children with all rights as fully grown members of a family]."*

> Matthew 22:37-40 AMP, *"And Jesus replied to him, 'YOU SHALL LOVE THE LORD YOUR GOD WITH ALL YOUR HEART, AND WITH ALL YOUR SOUL, AND WITH ALL YOUR MIND.' This is the first and greatest commandment. The second is like it, 'YOU SHALL LOVE YOUR NEIGHBOR AS YOURSELF [that is, unselfishly seek the best or higher good for others].' The whole Law and the [writings of the] Prophets depend on these two commandments."*

If followed and integrated correctly, the values of this book will empower you to be your best self. *Not in the cliché way people market these days, but fully empowered to fully focus on loving God and others— what we were created for, greatness.*

I pray that at least one chapter so far has spoken to you and encourages change. Finally, as we put all of this together, I will challenge you to think holistically by integrating the 5 concepts

(Recovery, Exercise, Nutrition, Mindfulness, and Faith) into the Body, Mind, and Spirit.

Reflect

How might your life look if you added prayer with faith to your daily situations, your injury or sickness, to those around you in need, or even into your business? What if you walked with faith that God is good and has your back in all situations, no matter what happens?

Chapter VII - Body, Mind, and Spirit

Romans 8:5 AMP *"For those who are living according to the flesh set their minds on the things of the flesh [which gratify the body], but those who are living according to the Spirit, [set their minds on] the things of the Spirit [His will and purpose]."*

How can you integrate all of this? Let's start with definitions. According to the Oxford Dictionary:

The Body is *"the physical structure of a person or an animal, including the bones, flesh, and organs."* One could say it's our physical person and what we host on this earth.

The Mind is *"the element of a person that enables them to be aware of the world and their experiences, to think, and to feel; the faculty of consciousness and thought."* One could say it's what we use to act, experience, and view the world as we know it.

The Spirit is *"the nonphysical part of a person which is the seat of emotions and character; the soul."* It's meant to be a reflection of God (we are created in His image to reflect His character) and makes us the unique person we are.

The purpose of this chapter, and why I want to bring the spirit and soul into the mix of wellness, is that if you're not careful, you may continue to separate them from your daily life and habits. As you can already begin to see, one does affect the other. So, let's continue bringing clarity to the topic.

Here's a visual of how they can relate to one another:

Body, Mind, and Spirit

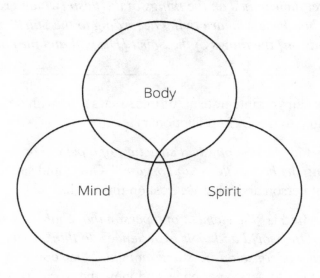

The picture above has been a clear vision of mine for a few years. Do you see the very center? When you unite purity in these three areas of your life, "you will see clearly." *In the purity of the body, mind, and spirit, I believe you see clearest.*

In Matthew 5:8 AMP Jesus states,

> *"Blessed [anticipating God's presence, spiritually mature] are the pure in heart [those with integrity, moral courage, and godly character], for they will see God."*

The Greek word *"see"* (horao) used in the Bible expands to the meaning *"to see with the eyes, to see with the mind, to perceive, to know, and become acquainted with by experience, to experience."* Also, another word for the *"face"* (paniym) of God in Hebrew is *"presence"* or *"wholeness of being"*.

It seems that purity goes a long way. When these dimensions of your self are pure and tended to, I believe (and have experienced myself) hearing, sensing, and loving God is at its easiest. There are no distractions. Nothing is separating you from the goodness of and sensitivity to the presence of God. Even if you aren't "perfect" in doing so (you don't live by works), God knows your heart and sees when you try with honest intention. There is grace.

However, there is also an opportunity for you here as an act of worship (Romans 12:1). *By intentionally setting the flesh aside, you can begin optimizing areas of your life for Him, to be transformed more and more daily into the image of Christ.* Imagine if you walked with this burning passion? If you walked with this conviction to tend to your body, mind, and spirit in a way that reflects how much He loves you, even cherishes you.

I believe you would operate with power and holiness through the Holy Spirit to a degree you've never experienced. You would see clearly what God has in store for you and walk-in a pure, unadulterated love that does not seek its own— daily. You have a powerful opportunity here.

You have been crafted by God. Let yourself never forget that.

So, how can you begin to walk this out? You must remember, you are ever connected as part of the human race, and even more interconnected as an individual person. It's complex and amazing how one part of you affects the other. Your posture can affect our mind and how you feel. Actions affect your thoughts, and your thoughts affect your actions. It's a never-ending cycle.

Because of this, I will touch back on the example of sugar (it's a good one). If you eat sugar, you know it can affect the chemicals in your brain and influence your mind. If your mind is affected, your body and spirit can be affected. Then as you carry on, your choices, behavior, and even your mood, can be influenced, which you may not even realize in the moment.

It's so subtle. Many of us don't even know what it feels like to feel our best.

Don't miss this. There is always a chain reaction. The actions you take hours before can dictate how you make current, daily choices. For many, over time, even anxiety or depression can begin to sink in when the actions we take aren't rooted with health in mind. This all works together, even integrating into your spirit, which I believe can in-turn limit your true potential to impact others. To make it plain and simple, you can come to a place of not walking in the Spirit as we are called to, which unfortunately is the common norm.

Ephesians 6:18 AMP, *"With all prayer and petition pray [with specific requests] at all times [on every occasion and in every season] in the Spirit, and with this in view, stay alert with all perseverance and petition [interceding in prayer] for all God's people."*

At the very least, poor health choices can cause inconsistency, which is the root of unproductivity for the Kingdom and the enemy's main goal. As a Believer, you are saved by grace, and the devil knows that. He has lost. All the enemy can do now is slow you down, burn you out, and/or distract you, keeping your focus on yourself. He can get you to a place where it's always about what you're doing, how you're feeling, what you want, and what you need.

Jesus didn't preach this kind of focus on self. Actually, He preached quite the opposite.

> Matthew 16:24 AMP, *"Then Jesus said to His disciples, "If anyone wishes to follow Me [as My disciple], he must deny himself [set aside selfish interests], and take up his cross [expressing a willingness to endure whatever may come] and follow Me [believing in Me, conforming to My example in living and, if need be, suffering or perhaps dying because of faith in Me]."*

Remember the revelation I had?

"If everything is a choice, including loving God, then eating foods that hinder our choices probably isn't a good idea."

As I talked about in chapter 4, these choices can include drinking, social media, and other habits that undermine your physical, mental, and spiritual health. You need to gain knowledge while learning moderation because pain, sickness, depression, and the like can all affect your spirituality as "distractions."

However, when you are stable, consistent, and working toward health in your physical body and mind, you will be better equipped to seek God and relationships with others with clarity, intention, and love. This in turn feeds into the spirit. Are you starting to see the connection? What if you learned to reset and refocus this holistic health as a priority?

This may help fuel your spirit rather than diminish it.

The following concept will help you practically integrate this into your life. In his book, *The Power of Less,* Leo Babauta writes about <u>most important tasks</u> (or MITs). This includes 2-4 tasks you accomplish first thing in the morning to start your day off right. When you accomplish these, as Babauta says himself, "no matter what, every day is a good day." I came up with an application you can do daily, working to tend to each area of your body, mind, and spirit. This is meant to be simple, easy, and doable to promote consistency.

Here's my example:

<u>Daily MITs</u>

1. Body

Exercise for 20 minutes.

2. Mind

Read 1 chapter of a book that challenges you and stimulates the mind.

3. Spirit

Pray and meditate on the Word in the *secret place* for 20 minutes.

All of this can be done in one hour or less. What if you consistently started every day like this? What would your life look like?

Visualize yourself walking in focus, freedom, health, and intention daily. You have the capability, and I will continue to reiterate, it starts with a foundation of wholeness to be at your best.

"Ok," you may say, "But I'm way off track. How do I even begin to get back?" or, "I'm not where I should be physically, mentally, or spiritually."

Boom. Here's a 5-step protocol I trust will get you back on the path:

1. Pray and repent

Most of us think repenting is to cry out and fall on our knees to God, but actually, the Greek word in the Bible for repent is "metanoia," meaning *"a change of mind"* (to change your direction).

As small as they may be, you need to acknowledge your faults and choices that have separated you from God's (hopeful) lifestyle for you and repent. You can "change your mind" to follow and trust Him, cutting distractions, and getting back on the path if you believe.

He will guide you. He is with you.

2. Practice self-compassion

We are all tempted. We all stumble. Be thankful for your awareness to recognize the roadblocks in your life and receive grace. The fact that you care is already a win!

"There is no such thing as failure, only feedback."
– John Berardi

Just keep moving forward. Use this time to learn and grow from the experience. Remember God's Word, *"You. Were. Made. For. Me."*

3. Take a small action

Easy does it. You don't have to solve the problem in one day. The best way to get back on track is to take a small action toward your goals. It could be as simple as taking one minute to breathe and reset. *Any small action toward your goals will create momentum and motivation, leading you to change.*

4. Set daily reminders

Once you are on a positive path, keep yourself reminded. Set up triggers or reminders to keep you on track and stay focused on the goal at hand. It could be a sticky note on your car dashboard, a daily phone reminder, or writing your vision on the bathroom mirror. *Whatever will help you to remember who and whose you are, where you are going, and to stay focused through the process.*

5. Reach out and find support

Community is key. You were built for it. It's important to let your family, friends, colleagues, and/or coach know your goals. Ask them to help you and support you along the way.

"Asking for help doesn't mean you are weak; it's actually
been shown to build trust."

- Brené Brown, *Dare to Lead*

If you follow this five-step process, I promise success over time. Don't give up. Failure happens. It's what makes us human. The question is, what will you do from there? *Just keep moving forward.*

Never forget you are here on Earth to love God and to reflect that love to others. You need to engage in your wellness, cutting out distractions to maximize your potential. In times like this, you have a great opportunity to manifest God in all you do, using the gifts you have been given for His glory and helping others. You can be the rock the world so desperately needs through Jesus Christ.

We each have a role to play, but will you commit?

Ephesians 5:15-16 AMP, *"Therefore see that you walk carefully [living life with honor, purpose, and courage; shunning those who tolerate and enable evil], not as the unwise, but as wise [sensible, intelligent, discerning people], making the very most of your time [on earth, recognizing and taking advantage of each opportunity and using it with wisdom and diligence], because the days are [filled with] evil."*

It all starts with you, your best, your selfless best, by walking in health and the freedom of knowing who you are, and what you are on earth to accomplish. I'm talking about leading your sphere of influence wherever God has planted you and trusting in the process. You can't always control the pain, sickness, and disease in your life and in the world, but you can do your best to *prevent* them and sow good seed. Beyond that, you must simply trust the will of God through faith, whether for healing or for growth.

> Galatians 6:7-8 AMP, *"Do not be deceived, God is not mocked; for whatever a man sows, this he will also reap. For the one who sows to his own flesh will from the flesh reap corruption, but the one who sows to the Spirit will from the Spirit reap eternal life. Let us not lose heart in doing good, for in due time we will reap if we do not grow weary. So then, while we have opportunity, let us do good to all people, and especially to those who are of the household of the faith."*

You reap what you sow. I believe in miracles. I believe in grace, healing, and the power of God, but you have to ask yourself, *"should God perform a miracle when I may just need to take better care of my body, mind, and spirit, sowing good seed?"* Without correction, you learn nothing.

Hebrews 12:4-10 AMP says this,

> *"You have not yet struggled to the point of shedding blood in your striving against sin; and you have forgotten the divine word of encouragement which is addressed to you as sons,*

> '*My son, do not make light of the discipline of the Lord,*
> *And do not lose heart and give up when you are corrected by him;*
> *For the Lord disciplines and corrects those whom He loves,*
> *And He punishes every son whom He receives and welcomes [to His heart].* '

You must submit to [correction for the purpose of] discipline; God is dealing with you as with sons; for what son is there whom his father does not discipline? Now if you are exempt from correction and without discipline, in which all [of God's children] share, then you are illegitimate children and not sons [at all]. Moreover, we have had earthly fathers who disciplined us, and we submitted and respected them [for training us]; shall we not much more willingly submit to the Father of spirits, and live [by learning from His discipline]? For our earthly fathers disciplined us for only a short time as seemed best to them; but He disciplines us for our good, so that we may share His holiness."

God loves you too much to allow you to wander blindly off the path as a son or daughter. You can take it personally and live with spite, or you can choose to live with wisdom and thankfulness. Diligence and stewardship toward the body as a temple go a long way. This is where good science meets faith.

In regard to prevention, research has shown an active lifestyle and healthy diet are linked to reducing your chance of cancer and other illnesses such as COVID-19, the flu, and similar viruses if you have a "robust" (or in other words, a well-rounded) immune system. Taking things even a notch further by integrating prayer, I believe you can maximize this prevention and protection with the armor of God. *In other words, being offensive in exercising your faith and walking in the spirit daily* (Ephesians 6:10-18).

Here is a visual by Precision Nutrition I use as a tool to help clients gain perspective and work through what they can and can't control. What would *you* write in each sphere?

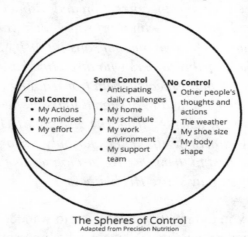

The Spheres of Control
Adapted from Precision Nutrition

I was having a discussion with a friend (shout out to Tyler), and we came up with another *360 Mindset*:

"Control what you can control. Pray for the rest". All you can control is what you sow. God can be trusted. He is just, good, and a healer, yet there is correction and corruption. You have free will, and you live in a broken, sinful world. You must not forget there will be many trials, but Christ has overcome them all. One could say you live in the beauty of chaos. I encourage you to take action, trusting and letting God bless the rest in HIS time.

James 1:2-4 AMP, *"Consider it nothing but joy, my brothers and sisters, whenever you fall into various trials. Be assured that the testing of your faith [through experience] produces endurance [leading to spiritual maturity, and inner peace]. And let endurance have its perfect result and do a thorough work, so that you may be perfect and completely developed [in your faith], lacking in nothing."*

John 16:33 AMP, *"I have told you these things, so that in Me you may have [perfect] peace. In the world you have tribulation and distress and suffering, but be courageous [be confident, be undaunted, be filled with joy]; I have overcome the world." [My conquest is accomplished, My victory abiding.]"*

You must abide in faith. It is your time to shine in the moments of trial by staying close to God and hearing His word. There's nothing stopping you if you set your needs aside and see trials as an opportunity to exude Jesus. Let me say, none of us are here by mistake. I'm writing this book during the COVID-19 pandemic and sense that Believers have a mighty purpose during this time. *You can make the deeper impact the world needs, if you believe in yourself (through Him) and let your actions reflect that belief.* You can control your choices, your diet, your activity, your recovery, your prayer time, how you respond, how you reach out, and much more.

Now, in order to do this and stay consistent, you must learn rest for the spirit. This also brings rest to the mind and body. I define this as receiving God's love in the secret place, daily.

Rest is the foundation of the spirit. Remember "devotional rest" in chapter 1? By His grace you are able to know God's Word (scripture), hear God's word (His voice), and have discernment for what is to come. You are to live by letting His presence dictate your circumstances and giving up your control. Not the other way around, keeping Christ and others from sharing your burdens (Galatians 6:2, Hebrews 4:15).

You need to learn to let God be God. The good things come when you let His grace and presence dictate your circumstances, not strive out of your own might. One could even say, strive outside of the Lord's will. I know for myself, I tend to get "ahead" of God. Here's one of my favorite quotes regarding resting in the Lord's will.

"Living presence conscious, not need conscious."

- Damon Thompson, Revivalist

When you seek God's presence and direction over the "solution," things open up for you that may not have otherwise if you had continued to strive and power through a circumstance. Only in devotional rest can you accomplish this way of living. In order to find this kind of rest, and hear His voice clearly, you will need to go into the "secret place." Shut your door. Become privately centered with the Lord and sit down. Listen. Invite His presence.

> Matthew 6:6 AMP, *"But when you pray, go into your most private room, close the door and pray to your Father who is in secret, and your Father who sees [what is done] in secret will reward you."*

Scripture shows us you can walk into the throne room of grace, boldly. *He loves you and created you for this very reason, to spend time with you, allowing you to walk in grace and abundance by reflecting His image.* Not because you strive but because you are His and rest in that truth daily, no matter what.

> Hebrews 4:15-16 AMP, *"For we do not have a High Priest who is unable to sympathize and understand our weaknesses and temptations, but One who has been tempted [knowing exactly how it feels to be human] in every respect as we are, yet without [committing any] sin.*

Therefore let us [with privilege] approach the throne of grace [that is, the throne of God's gracious favor] with confidence and without fear, so that we may receive mercy [for our failures] and find [His amazing] grace to help in time of need [an appropriate blessing, coming just at the right moment]."

2 Corinthians 3:17-18 AMP, *"Now the Lord is the Spirit, and where the Spirit of the Lord is, there is liberty [emancipation from bondage, true freedom]. And we all, with unveiled face, continually seeing as in a mirror the glory of the Lord, are progressively being transformed into His image from [one degree of] glory to [even more] glory, which comes from the Lord, [who is] the Spirit."*

As an illustration of this principle, let's visit a passage in Luke to remind you how God can work in your life, not by you constantly staying busy, but by devotional rest with the One who made you— allowing grace to triumph.

Luke 9:12-17 AMP, *"Now the day was ending, and the twelve [disciples] came and said to Him, 'Send the crowd away, so that they may go into the surrounding villages and countryside and find lodging, and get provisions; because here we are in an isolated place.' But He said to them, 'You give them something to eat.' They said, 'We have no more than five loaves and two fish—unless perhaps we go and buy food for all these people.' (For there were about 5,000 men.) And He said to His disciples, 'Have them sit down to eat in groups of about fifty each.' They did so, and had them all sit down. Then He took the five loaves and the two fish, and He looked up to heaven [and gave thanks] and blessed them, and broke them and kept giving them to the disciples to set before the crowd. They all ate and were [completely]*

> *satisfied; and the broken pieces which they had left over were [abundant and were] picked up—twelve baskets full."*

The miracle in this passage was an act of devotional rest. Instead of running to the store, Jesus had them sit down. You only find this kind of fulfillment in the secret place, at the feet of Jesus, resting at the feet of the One we call King and giving thanks. This is a kingdom mentality, counterintuitive to the way the world thinks and behaves, fully trusting in God who is your good Father.

Letting God tend to your spirit, growing and learning to love in His presence, reading the word and being trained for where He wants you in this world— this is "true rest." There are people in your life who are there for you, but God is there for you even more so, to an infinite degree (Ephesians 3:18). He promises to ultimately take care of you, and all your needs (Matthew 10:29). Sometimes all you have to do is sit down and *receive*.

If you would like to dive deeper in your relationship with God, there's a book called *Secrets of the Secret Place* by Bob Sorge that I recommend. I am just touching on the secret place and how it is related to your spirit and wellness, but he takes it much further into how you can seek God and ignite your personal relationship with Him.

Below are 3 practical components I believe make up the secret place, just to get you started:

1. Prayer

Practicing gratitude, praying for others according to God's will, and praying out your cares to God.

> *"Therefore, confess your sins to one another [your false steps, your offenses], and pray for one another,*

that you may be healed and restored. The heartfelt and persistent prayer of a righteous man (believer) can accomplish much [when put into action and made effective by God—it is dynamic and can have tremendous power]."

James 5:16 AMP

2. Reading

Meditating (or mindfully reading and taking every word into consideration) on the Word of God.

> *"This Book of the Law shall not depart from your mouth, but you shall read [and meditate on] it day and night, so that you may be careful to do [everything] in accordance with all that is written in it; for then you will make your way prosperous, and then you will be successful."*

Joshua 1:8 AMP

3. Waiting on the Lord

Resting and listening to what God is saying during your season. Seeking direction, clarity, love, and hope from the Father.

> *"But those who wait for the Lord [who expect, look for, and hope in Him]*
> *Will gain new strength and renew their power;*
> *They will lift up their wings [and rise up close to God] like eagles [rising toward the sun];*
> *They will run and not become weary,*
> *They will walk and not grow tired."*

Isaiah 40:31 AMP

These three actions stoke the flame of the Spirit inside of you, igniting passion for the Lord and serving others while bringing true rest to your weary soul.

I challenge you today, review your notes taken throughout this book and meditate on them. Pray, seek, and ask God to reveal your purpose and the next steps in all of this to you. Remember to *listen*. He longs to spend time with you and reveal His wisdom. Without true rest, this cannot happen.

> James 1:5 AMP, *"If any of you lacks wisdom [to guide him through a decision or circumstance], he is to ask of [our benevolent] God, who gives to everyone generously and without rebuke or blame, and it will be given to him."*

Ask with faith... I know He will answer!

Reflect

Out of the Body, Mind, and Spirit, is there an area of your life you find yourself neglecting more than the others? What can you do to strengthen it? How will you implement this in your everyday life?

Conclusion

1 Peter 4:1-2 AMP, *"Therefore, since Christ suffered in the flesh [and died for us], arm yourselves [like warriors] with the same purpose [being willing to suffer for doing what is right and pleasing God], because whoever has suffered in the flesh [being like-minded with Christ] is done with [intentional] sin [having stopped pleasing the world], so that he can no longer spend the rest of his natural life living for human appetites and desires, but [lives] for the will and purpose of God."*

Your potential is endless, but to fully enable growth, you must first find your balance in body, mind, and spirit, building a healthy foundation in yourself that others can abide in and look up to as a leader.

You must continually work toward a consistent foundation of wellness and wholeness, living life to the fullest. Through this, there's a freedom and opportunity for fulfillment like no other. This won't come from doing what's easy. The days are evil, and the world is in opposition to the mind of Christ. Only by living against the grain can you break through. Will you join me?

At the end of the day, *transformation* is about identity, remembering who you are, as a child of God first and foremost. There is everlasting life when you lay down your own, for both the present and the life to come.

Matthew 10:39 AMP, *"Whoever finds his life [in this world] will [eventually] lose it [through death], and whoever loses his life [in this world] for My sake will find it [that is, life with Me for all eternity]."*

If you are going to take away one thing from what I've written, I would want you to know you are created for so much more than you may realize. Yes, you! *In order to maximize this truth in your life, however, you are going to need to apply consistent action toward true health and wellness; integrating the concepts of these pages with self-discipline, persistence, endurance, and faith.* You were made in His image, and the time is now to let Christ shine in every area of your life. It's a life of selfless giving, yet you will be made whole through the process. I have a burning passion to see all who believe live up to the potential for which they were created.

I feel God's heart break over the potential not lived in every one of us.

Ephesians 1:18-21 AMP states,

> *"And [I pray] that the eyes of your heart [the very center and core of your being] may be enlightened [flooded with light by the Holy Spirit], so that you will know and cherish the hope [the divine guarantee, the confident expectation] to which He has called you, the riches of His glorious inheritance in the saints (God's people), and [so that you will begin to know] what the immeasurable and unlimited and surpassing greatness of His [active, spiritual] power is in us who believe. These are in accordance with the working of His mighty strength which He produced in Christ when He raised Him from the dead and seated Him at His own right hand in the heavenly places, far above all rule and authority and power and dominion [whether angelic or human], and [far above] every name that is named [above every title that can be conferred], not only in this age and world but also in the one to come."*

No longer can you continue to neglect the temple of God within and the power you now possess through Christ. You must nurture and tend to it through intentional recovery, exercise, nutrition, and mindfulness, while cultivating and integrating faith to build a foundation of growth and impact. *Wholeness is about hitting every angle, and in this you can maximize your true, God-given potential.* The way of living you're called to may not look like the world, but you're called to be different. You're called to impact the world from a different position, centered in Christ, no matter where God has planted you.

You can be a schoolteacher and have impact. You can be a night security guard and have impact. You can be a stay-at-home parent and have impact. You can be in school, and unsure of your first career and have an impact. It's ok. It doesn't matter what you do, it's how you do it that makes a difference. Let those who have ears, hear.

Mark 4:23-25 NASB, " *'If anyone has ears to hear, let him hear.' And He was saying to them, 'Take care what you listen to. By your standard of measure it will be measured to you; and more will be given you besides. For whoever has, to him more shall be given; and whoever does not have, even what he has shall be taken away from him.'"*

Matthew 11:12-15 NASB, *"From the days of John the Baptist until now the kingdom of heaven suffers violence, and violent men take it by force. For all the prophets and the Law prophesied until John. And if you are willing to accept it, John himself is Elijah who was to come. He who has ears to hear, let him hear."*

Jesus talks about an opportunity here. Will you rise to the occasion of wholeheartedness (zealous passion for God), embracing your greatness? Or will you miss out on the life of impact God has destined you for?

> *"You can stumble into forgiveness, but you can't stumble into wholeheartedness."*

- Mike Bickle, Founder of International House of Prayer

You are called to be a doer of the word, not merely a hearer. You are called to love others, seek the will of God, live out the gospel of Christ, and tend to your body as a temple of God. I urge you to no longer conform to the world, letting it identify you. Instead, cut distractions, continue to find your identity in Christ, and be the light of the world. It needs you, and God wants to use you.

James 1:22-24 AMP, *"But prove yourselves doers of the word, and not merely hearers who delude themselves. For if anyone is a hearer of the word and not a doer, he is like a man who looks at his natural face in a mirror; for once he has looked at himself and gone away, he has immediately forgotten what kind of person he was."*

1 Peter 1:4-8 NASB, *"For by these He has granted to us His precious and magnificent promises, so that by them you may become partakers of the divine nature, having escaped the corruption that is in the world by lust. Now for this very reason also, applying all diligence, in your faith supply moral excellence, and in your moral excellence, knowledge, and in your knowledge, self-control, and in your self-control, perseverance, and in your perseverance, godliness, and in your godliness, brotherly kindness, and in your brotherly kindness, love. For if these qualities are yours and are increasing, they render you neither useless nor unfruitful in the true knowledge of our Lord Jesus Christ."*

So, find your team, write down your goals, be easy on yourself, enjoy the process, and never forget who you are. *You were created for greatness, and it starts now.* I challenge you to share this book with 5 people you know could benefit by reading these chapters. If you decide to try the **21 Day: Dopamine Fast,** I hope you can use the guidelines and encouragement in this book to stay centered in Him through the process.

Trust. Listen. Hear. God wants to speak to you during this time, and I want to see your greatness begin to shine throughout this next season. Remember your 5 Whys in Chapter 1— your true reason for reading this book.

I pray that by this time, you're able to clearly see each and every value in recovery, exercise, nutrition, mindfulness, and faith that speaks to you. Meditate, identify, and apply ways you can add to your life through these. There is always more to learn and room for growth for those who want to be great. So, find what works for you, trust your passions, and stay true to God's love.

As a Christian body, it is our time to unite and encourage one another to pursue this holistic, faith-based health I call wholeness.

I further pray for peace and protection over you and your household. Keep moving forward and keep the faith. I truly care for you and believe God will guide your path as you continue to abide in Him. There is hope, healing, and health in this. God bless.

John 1:2 AMP, *"Beloved, I pray that in every way you may succeed and prosper and be in good health [physically], just as [I know] your soul prospers [spiritually]."*

Reflect

What was your biggest breakthrough or takeaway after reading this book? If you'd like, share your answer with Jackson by emailing 360wellnessllc@gmail.com *or leave us a review.*

THANK YOU SO MUCH FOR READING

YOU WERE CREATED FOR GREATNESS

If this content helped you in anyway, please leave an online review on Amazon or Barnes and Noble to help more readers discover their greatness.

About The Author

"God loves and has goodness and rest for each and every one of us. I want to share that through what I do as a writer and a coach." –Jackson Hale

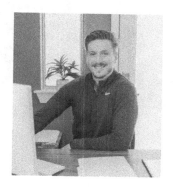

Jackson Hale is the founder of 360wellness, a hybrid non-profit Christian Wellness Center located in Carlsbad, California. With a background in physical therapy, fitness training, and health coaching, he has a vision to start a new concept of healthcare— one that improves health for the body, mind, and spirit through faith-based and practical applications. Jackson's passion is to work with all people, empower churches, and serve the less fortunate at no cost. His goal is to make a global impact as a non-profit organization and motivate others to find the greatness they were created for. His credentials include: B.S. Applied Exercise Science (Physical Therapy focus), CAMTC Licensed Massage Therapist, Precision Nutrition Lvl 1 Coach, and NASM Corrective Exercise Specialist/Certified Personal Trainer.

Learn more about Jackson and 360wellness
https://the360wellness.com

CPSIA information can be obtained
at www.ICGtesting.com
Printed in the USA
FSHW011329240421
80702FS